First Edition

Published by WILLOWRAVENCREST LLC

ISBN 979-8-234-15580-1

Printed in the United States of America

CURIOUS ATROCITIES

The Dark Side of Obscured History

Welcome to the Dark Side

An Invitation to Investigate and Wander the Unknown

WILLOW RAVENCREST

DISCLAIMER

This book explores difficult and often disturbing chapters of history, including medical abuse, government experimentation, pseudoscience, and other sensitive subjects. Reader discretion is advised.

While every effort has been made to present accurate information based on available historical records and credible sources, history is inherently complex and subject to interpretation. Sources sometimes contradict one another, and new information may emerge over time.
The accounts presented here reflect the author's best understanding at the time of writing.

The links and QR codes included in this book were functional at the time of publication. The author does not own, control, or endorse external websites and is not responsible for their content or any changes that may occur after publication.

This book is not intended as a definitive historical record, nor should it replace independent research. Instead an invitation to question, explore, and think critically about the stories we are told.
Readers are strongly encouraged to examine multiple sources, consider differing perspectives and draw their own conclusions.

WILLOW RAVENCREST

Dedications

To my Grandmother, who always pushed me to go further than I believed possible and taught me to question my own limits.

To my Grandfather, who raised me to be fiercely independent. He never held me back for being a girl and always welcomed me into the heart of the work—tools in hand, right beside him.

To the Dear Friends I have loved and lost to the sands of time. You taught me that life is ever-evolving and that I am far braver than I often believe.

To my Mom Thank You for helping teach me how nieve I was as a child. Thank You for always being there for my kids.

To my Dad, who showed me what hard work, perseverance, and dedication truly look like.

To my Spouse Thank You for filling my last ten years full of laughter and a love I never thought possible. Thank you for busting your ass every day for our family.

And most of all, to my children.

You all have changed my entire world in the blink of an eye and set me on the path that ultimately led to these pages. Every challenge, every lesson, every question, and every discovery brought me here.

Thank you for shaping who I am.

Willow Ravencrest

Epigraph

"The important thing is not to stop questioning.

Curiosity has its own reason for existing."

— Albert Einstein

"History is a set of lies agreed upon."

— Napoleon Bonaparte

"It is easier to deceive people than to convince them they have been deceived."

— Mark Twain

The greatest atrocities are rarely recognized as atrocities while they are happening.

They are justified.

Defended.

Explained away.

Only later do we ask how anyone could have believed them.

This book begins with that question.

May any questions that arise lead to curiosity.

Willow Ravencrest

TABLE OF CONTENTS

PART IV

State Power, Government Abuse & Cover-Ups

PREFACE

I have always been a skeptic. Even as a child, I asked too many questions. This habit frequently got me into trouble in school, but it also opened doors in my mind that many people preferred to keep closed. The unknown has fascinated me for as long as I can remember—whether it was hidden corners of history, the complexities of the human mind, or the strange behaviors of the natural world.

After years of struggling with infertility and being told I would never have children—or even live past thirty—I was given a chance to defy the odds. With the help of the incredible Stork Program in Nashville, Tennessee, and a wonderful OB, I became a mother. I made the decision to leave the workforce and become a stay-at home mom.

What began as a fight for survival became one of the greatest blessings of my life. Raising my children, and later experiencing both homeschooling and public education, gave me a front-row seat to how the next generation is taught—and how much of what we call "history" and "truth" is carefully curated.

Watching my children learn, I became increasingly frustrated by how often uncomfortable facts were softened, simplified, or omitted entirely. The more I researched, the clearer it became that many stories from our past are far more complicated than the versions most of us inherit.

This book was born from that frustration—and from a deep belief that we cannot grow as individuals or as a society if we refuse to examine our mistakes. It is not a book of final answers. It is an invitation.

An invitation to follow the questions.

An invitation to explore uncomfortable truths.

An invitation to wander into the forgotten corners of history and decide for yourself what they mean.

Some of these stories may make you angry. Some may break your heart. Others may leave you wondering how many of today's accepted truths will one day be viewed with the same disbelief we now reserve for bloodletting, phrenology, and countless other ideas once considered unquestionable.

If this book makes you uncomfortable, good.

If it makes you curious, even better.

And if it inspires you to dig deeper, challenge assumptions, and think for yourself, then it has accomplished exactly what it was meant to do.

Welcome to the rabbit holes.

Welcome to the dark side.

WILLOW RAVENCREST

INTRODUCTION

History can teach us a lot. It shows us where we come from, how we got here as a human race, and how small moments can completely reshape the world. But if you look just beyond what you're supposed to learn — past the clean, simplified version taught in textbooks — you'll often find something far more unsettling.

The forgotten corners. The uncomfortable truths. The moments that were rewritten, buried, or deliberately ignored. That's exactly what this book is about.

There are key moments in history that completely changed the way we think, live, and view the world. We will explore the parts of history that challenge what we think we know. Some truths stayed hidden for years — even centuries — only to be uncovered long after the damage was done.

You hear the stories all the time: great inventors and thinkers mocked or shunned in their lifetime, only to be celebrated after they were gone. What we call "settled fact" today can be disproven tomorrow. Scientists declare something safe, only to later list all the ways it can harm or even kill us. One doctor gives a firm diagnosis while another says the complete opposite. The debate never seems to end.

How much of what we currently believe will be proven wrong in the next ten years?

As the years pile up, we keep discovering that much of what we once accepted as true is no longer accurate. Our understanding of the world is constantly evolving. Right and wrong, safe and dangerous, history and science — these lines are far more fluid than most people are comfortable admitting.

How much do we really know about anything? Is "truth" sometimes just a matter of perspective? And how often do we mistake confidence for certainty?

These days the world feels like it's changing faster than ever. In this book, you will encounter many of those shifts — some short and almost strange, others deep, heavy, and profoundly disturbing. A few topics may feel controversial. I've woven in my own thoughts and reflections alongside the research, but I encourage you not to take my word for it. If you're uncertain about anything you read, dive down the rabbit hole for yourself, explore the sources, and draw your own conclusions

I'll be honest: there was real hesitation in writing certain parts of this book. There are pieces of our history that many would prefer stayed buried. They don't paint a flattering picture of humanity. They're not the simple, clean, comfortable version taught in schools. They show the ugly truth, but I believe that in order to learn from our mistakes, we must face them.

History is doomed to repeat itself if we only ever examine the polished, sanitized version. This book is my attempt to shine a light into those shadows

If you decide to continue reading, I hope it encourages you to dig a little deeper into everything you think you know. I hope you learn things you've never heard before. Every day is an opportunity to expand your mind and challenge your reality. My hope is that this book leaves you seeing the world with new eyes.

Before you turn the page, I want you to pause and ask yourself honestly: Are you ready for what's in these pages?

Some of these topics are uncomfortable. Some are disturbing. Some things, once seen, cannot be unseen. At the bottom of this introduction you'll find the full list of topics covered. Please think carefully before going deeper. Some of what you read may stay with you for a long time.

Now, if you're ready… let's step into these rabbit holes together and see what we discover.

I cannot promise that every single "fact" in this book is 100% accurate. History is messy. Many sources cite different details. Some facts come from studies and are only approximations. In some cases, the full data is missing or has been lost to time. Please keep all of this in mind as you read. This book is only meant to give you a glimpse into these topics. I encourage each and everyone of you to dig into them for yourselves. Throughout history, some of humanity's greatest mistakes were made by people who were absolutely certain they were right.

Curious Atrocities Introduction

Below is the complete list of topics covered in this book:

Trephination- Phrenology- Cure for left-handedness- Bloodletting- Homo Conversion Therapy- Mass/Female Hysteria- Moral Insanity- Witch Trials/Witch Hunts- Satanic Panic- Recovered Memory Therapy- Ignaz Semmelweis & Handwashing- Smoking Advertised as Healthy- The Radium Girls- Transorbital Lobotomy of Walter FreemII-Mental disorders/Asylums and Treatments- Drapetomania-Sluggish Schizophrenia- Gulf War Syndrome- Forced Sterilization of Native Americans- Tuskegee Syphilis experiments- Eugenics Program- CIA MKUltra- Operation Paperclip / Overcast / Cover-upof Unit 731

PART I

Curious Pseudoscience

&

Early Misunderstandings

Trephination

Also known as Trepantation or making a burr hole, involves drilling a hole in your skull exposing the brain. It was used to treat all kinds of things from falls, hunting accidents, injuries to the brain, spiritual purposes, epilepsy, and even mental illnesses. The main goals were usually to relieve pressure from skull fractures/brain swelling or for ritual/spiritual reasons. In some societies it was used in attempts to treat mental illness or behavioral problems.

At one burial site in France dated to 6500 BCE, 40 out of 120 skulls found had Trephination holes. Many archaeological studies show survival rates for prehistoric trephination were actually quite high (often 50–90% depending on the site and time period), with evidence of healing around the holes. Trephination dates all the way back to 7,000-10,000 years ago.

The technique is still used today in a limited way to drill under finger/toe nails to relieve pain associated with Subungual Hematoma. Since the early 1960s voluntary trepanation has been performed on people interested in enhancing mental power and well-being.

Trephination was a risky ancient surgery that had some practical applications that we still use to this day. We took methods that were once used to bring real harm to people, to help people today. How much will change 15 years from now? Would you drill a hole in your skull to achieve spiritual enlightenment?

PHRENOLOGY

Phrenology is the concept that the brain is composed of different organs. When the organ is used more, it grows larger, which is supposedly why people had different head shapes. They thought that those shapes could be measured and it would tell them about that person's personality, strengths, weaknesses, and potential career possibilities and mental traits.

Phrenology influenced early psychiatry/psychology in the early 19th century. A list of "brain organs" was put out by German physician Franz Joseph Gall in 1796. It was believed there were 27 "brain organs" and depending on how big or small those bumps, determined who you were as a person. A Phrenologist would feel your head using their knowledge of the chart of brain organs, to determine the natural weaknesses/strengths, or personality of the person they are touching.

In 1819, ten years after he started his work he published The Anatomy and Physiology of the Nervous System in General, and of the Brain in Particular, with Observations upon the possibility of ascertaining the several Intellectual and Moral Dispositions of Man and Animal, by the configuration of the Heads.

Some of Gall's doctrinal principles which comprise the intellectual basis of phrenology:

The Brain is the organ of the mind

The brain is not a homogeneous unity, but an aggregate of mental organs with specific functions

The cerebral organs are topographically localized

Other things being equal, the relative size of any particular mental organ is indicative of the power or strength of that organ. Since the skull ossifies over the brain during infant development, external craniological means could be used to diagnose the internal states of the mental characters.

Through careful observation and some extensive experimentation Gall believed he had established a relationship between aspects of character or faculties with precise organs in the brain.

American brothers Orson Squire Fowler (1809-1887) and Lorenzo Niles Fowler (1811-1896) were leading phrenologists of their time. Lorenzo gained fame in England with his phrenology head, which became a symbol of phrenology. Lorenzo's head was used by a lot of phrenologists to "diagnose" patients. Orson, with associates Nelson Sizer and Samuel Robert Wells, ran Fowlers & Wells a phrenological business and publishing house in New York City. Both of the brothers' works on phrenology are displayed in museums today.

Stereotypes were common with phrenology, one example is women who have heads that are large in the back, or lower foreheads, were deemed no good at arts or sciences but very good for care of children or religion. Ladies, feel your head. Does it fit you? At one point in time, that could have been used as a diagnosis for you had our understanding of the brain not evolved. Perhaps the most troubling part of phrenology wasn't that it was wrong. It was that so many people accepted it as fact. Once an idea gains the appearance of science, people often stop questioning it.

In the USA in 1834 a professor of Anatomy at Rutgers Medical College defended the idea of Phrenology. By the 1940s it had largely lost credibility and is now deemed pseudoscience. Phrenology was once treated as an established fact. We all know differently today.

THE "CURE" FOR LEFT-HANDEDNESS

Left-handedness has a long, weird history of being treated like something abnormal, unlucky, or even straight-up evil.

In ancient Rome the word for left is sinister, yep you heard that right. A few Latin terms for left-handed weren't any better: laevus meant clumsy or foolish, and scaevus meant unlucky, perverse, unfortunate. They really didn't like lefties back then.

Fast forward to medieval times, and it got even darker. Being left-handed was often seen as a sign you were cursed or possessed by the devil. In some cases, it could get you accused of witchcraft. For centuries, left-handed people dealt with suspicion, cruelty, and discrimination. They were blocked from certain jobs, from becoming priests, and sometimes even basic respect. Can you imagine being called "unclean", "cursed" or "evil" just for using your left hand?

People threw salt over their left shoulder to ward off bad luck. "Right-hand man" is a very common saying implying the important and trusted person is to your right. It's everywhere! Many believed God was right-handed, which made the left hand the domain of Satan. These beliefs were so prevalent that families went to great lengths to force their children to use their right hand. They didn't want to be shunned or have to deal with all of the accusations.

Cesare Lombroso is an Italian criminologist, phrenologist, physician, eugenicist, and founder of the Italian school of criminology. Through his observation of criminals and sex workers he hypothesized a connection between being left-handed and being a criminal or having degenerative behaviour.

He also pushed the idea that being left-handed leads to disabilities by linking left-handedness with neurodegeneration and alcoholism. In his later years he did a series of research studies grouping being left handed with autoimmune diseases and psychiatric disorders.

Curing Left-handedness is laughable in our day but back in the early 1900s it was taken very seriously. People had to endure all kinds of treatments/cures for simply being left handed. It was commonly believed that left-handedness was linked to stuttering, criminality, cognitive impairment and at times a sin. Lefties out there, be thankful if you never had to experience any of it. I'm sure there are a few of our elders who could talk about it.

The treatments were meant to convert someone, usually kids from writing with their left hand to using their right hand. For generations, countless children were told that a natural part of who they were was wrong and needed to be corrected. Today it seems absurd. It raises an uncomfortable question: what accepted practices of our own time will future generations view the same way? They would use methods such as tying the left hand behind the back, corporal punishment, and shaming. Ironically it was found that all of the things they did to "help/ cure" it did the very thing they claimed leaving it alone would do.

Promotions for the cure to left-handedness were boosted all over even down to the tiny town newspapers and pamphlets. I hold an article from the 1920s that was found on a wall in an 1800s home. It talks about the "cure for left-handedness." Today this theory is laughed at in social circles and heavily frowned upon by professionals. How many times has mankind been wrong about so many other small simple things like this? How many do we really know about? How many have been lost to time or forgotten? What other cures do we have now that could be deemed "crazy" or questionable in the next decade or two?

Would you have believed this if you lived then?

Bloodletting

Ancient times–19th century

It was thought the human body was made of four humors: black bile, yellow bile, blood and phlegm. Bloodletting was a cure for restoring appetite, improving sleep, curing disease, remedy for plague, epilepsy, smallpox, hypertension, headaches, inflammation, fever, asthma, pneumonia, mental illness, vomiting, menstrual issues and a host of other deadly maladies. Granted all of those different ailments were layered on over the years.

In the early times of bloodletting they used animal teeth, sharp thorns and similar items that were deemed “sharp”. Egyptians are believed to have practiced bloodletting, there are two references to scarification (cutting/etching the skin to make permanent scars) in the Ebers Papyrus. It became well established in Greece as Hippocrates, the father of medicine, recommended bloodletting especially at the elbows and knees.

Male patients suffering from smallpox would have leeches applied to their scrotum to help with swollen testicles. Leeches were often used in bloodletting simply because they are capable of ingesting around ten times their own weight. Doctors would place the leech on the body, encouraging it to bite the patient, while watching it grow in size the more blood it sucked from the body. Gentlemen, would you willingly let a leech bite your scrotum?

Cupping was another attempt at bloodletting. A small incision was made and a suction cup was used to draw out the blood. Following a papal decree in 1163 which prohibited priests from bloodletting. The practice was adopted by barbers, who became known as barber-surgeons. The red stripe on those well known barber poles came from the blood-stained towels that dominated their workplace. Bloodletting was said to be beneficial to one's health to do it a few times a year.

Benjamin Rush was an American physician, political leader, signer of the Declaration of Independence, and member of the Continental Congress. He was also an avid believer in bloodletting and purging as medical treatments. French conqueror Napoleon was one of the few survivors of bloodletting. It was so traumatic he later reportedly stated "medicine is the science of murderers."

In December 1799 President George Washington was diagnosed with a cold and mild hoarseness. Two days later he was worse and called for his aides and doctors. Washington endured purgatives, emetics as well as having half his blood drained. The combination of treatments likely contributed to shock and a dangerous drop in blood pressure, ultimately ending the life of the nation's first president. Ladies and gentlemen, were you taught that in history class?

Veterinarian J. Thompson, a British veterinarian, was among the first to publicly challenge the practice in 1792. Bloodletting gradually lost credibility throughout the mid-1800s as germ theory and advances in physiology gained acceptance.

What science or medical practice accepted today might future generations view the same way we now view bloodletting?

While modern medicine still uses controlled blood removal in certain circumstances for specific conditions, the practice survives in some cultures and spiritual traditions as well.

WANT TO DIG DEEPER?

The following pages contain links to museum collections, archives, historical photographs, public records, documentaries, and other resources related to each section of this book.

Scan the QR code or type the web address to continue your investigation.

TREPHINATION

Resource

https://commons.wikimedia.org/w/index.php?curid=26657586

PHRENOLOGY

Resource

https://publicdomainreview.org/collection/phrenology-diagrams-from-vaught-s-practical-character-reader-1902/

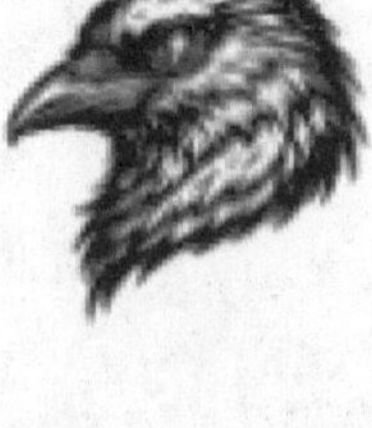

PART II

Social & Cultural Enforcement

Homo Conversion Therapy

Richard von Krafft-Ebing, a German-Austrian psychiatrist and a founder of scientific sexology. His work in 1886 Psychopathia Sexualis had a discussion of methods for curing homosexuality through hypnosis. Albert von Schrenck-Notzing, a German psychiatrist, bragged at a conference, claimed that through hypnosis and taking the patient (gay guy) to a brothel, he had cured his gayness.

In an analysis done in the 1920s it was assumed homosexuality was pathological and attempts to treat it were necessary. Eugen Steinach, an Austrian physiologist and pioneer in endocrinology theorized the testes secretion was testosterone. He experimented and transplanted the testes of a male guinea pig into a female. It resulted in the female developing male behavior like mounting the partner. This theory led to the transplant of testicles of straight men into gay men to change their sexual preference. At times it even led to castration. In 1923 Steinach commissioned a film on his work where he transplanted one half of a testicle of a heterosexual man into the groin of a homosexual man. He was attempting to change the sexual proclivities of the homosexual.

Robert Galbraith Heath, a psychiatrist in New Orleans, is seen as a pioneer in the technique, a form of electroshock therapy. Electrodes were implanted directly into the brain along with hiring prostitutes and playing heterosexual porn to "change" the sexual orientation of gay men. He adamantly claimed his techniques could turn gay men straight.

When it comes to the camps a lot of the information is rather hard to access. If you grew up in this era you remember the clips all over the media. The most retold story is of Garrad Conley who handed over his handbook from his time at "Love in Action" out of Memphis Tennessee. While compelling it is still only one man's story from one camp. These camps were spread throughout multiple countries.

Throughout history there have been many "treatments" for homosexuality such as bladder washing, rectal massage, castration, hypnosis, confrontation therapy, conversion camps, Aversion therapy, drugs, lobotomies, hormone therapy, Masturbatory/Orgasmic Reconditioning, rewarding for heterosexual behavior, beating/isolation recommended to parents for "nonconforming" behaviors and more. If you're not certain what some of those are I would highly recommend looking them up especially aversion therapy.

These were beliefs/treatments that lasted for decades, from the 1920s into the early 2000s. While we no longer openly practiced most of these methods today, homosexuals have remained heavy targets of discrimination and violence. There was a period where hate crimes against homosexuals appeared to decline, but in recent years new debates surrounding gender identity, medical interventions, and the treatment of minors have created fresh cultural divisions.

Much like previous generations, people today often feel strongly convinced that their position is the correct one. This is a tricky topic for anyone to cover anymore. Each side is so opposed to the other. Somewhere beneath the noise, certainty, and emotion surrounding the issue lies a truth that future generations may understand differently than we do today. This has been going on for over a century in some form or another. Do you honestly think there will be a resolution any time soon? What will people believe in even five years? I sometimes wonder how future generations will judge some of today's medical interventions involving children and adolescents. History repeatedly reminds us that treatments once considered compassionate, progressive, or scientifically settled have later been reevaluated—or even condemned. Which of today's certainties will tomorrow's historians question?

Mass/Female Hysteria

In psychology and sociology, Mass Hysteria is a phenomenon that spreads a collective illusion of threats through a population and society, whether real or fake. In medicine it is used to describe the same hysterical physical symptoms by one or more people. Throughout our history there have been many different types of hysteria that have at times taken over towns. Leaving those around wondering what was happening.

The witch trials from 1450-1750, with the worst years occurring between 1580-1630. People believed witches working with Satan were out to do the devil's bidding. The dancing plague of 1518 where a case of dancing mania occurred in Strasbourg, Alsace. Numerous people in the town broke out in dance for days on end. In December of 1688 in England and parts of Wales during the Glorious Revolution, at least 19 different counties took up arms preparing to resist a non-existent group of marauding Irishmen. The mass panic was caused by false reports that Irish soldiers were burning and massacring English towns.

The Salem Witch Trials 1692-1693 in Massachusetts is a prime example of mass hysteria. A series of hearings resulted in the execution of citizens for the crimes of witchcraft. In Würzburg, Germany 1749, an outbreak of trance behavior, squirming and screaming in a nunnery resulted in the death of a suspected witch. The medieval vampire scares. People went to great lengths to bury their dead so if they came back as vampires they would be trapped or die.

“War of the Worlds” radio broadcast 1938, Orson Welles radio convinced thousands of Americans they were under a deadly Martian attack. The resulting mass hysteria in 1976 Mount Pleasant, Mississippi caused one third of the school's 900 students to stay home out of fear of being “hexed” after 15 students fell to the ground writhing. 1981 Clown hysteria panic starting in Boston, Massachusetts, spreading throughout the United States and Canada. Reports of children seeing evil clowns often engaging in frightening behavior.

As you can see from the examples above, episodes of mass hysteria have appeared across cultures, countries, and centuries. How many of these panics or outbreaks had you heard of before today?

Below is a closer look at female hysteria, sometimes referred to as the "wandering womb" theory. Yes, you read that correctly. For centuries, many people genuinely believed a woman's uterus could move throughout her body and cause physical and emotional distress wreaking havoc. It was a very real and common medical diagnosis for women as far back as 1900 BC in Egypt and Greece. It was said to have a pretty wide array of symptoms, anxiety, shortness of breath, nervousness, irritability, fainting, exaggerated and impulsive sexual desires, heaviness in the abdomen, loss of appetite for food and sex, fluid retention, insomnia, sexually impulsive behaviors, tears and laughter, yawning, difficulty swallowing, chest pain, delirium, cold extremities, abundant and clear urine. That was a lot, anyone else felt exhausted after reading all of that.

This was an "illness/problem" in women for centuries. Beliefs about its symptoms and treatments varied throughout the ages. Women, how many times would you have been diagnosed with hysteria by now? Men, how many times would you have been? Charles Lepois (Caroli Pisonis) and Thomas Willis argued in the 17th century that hysteria could stem from the brain, not the uterus, therefore being able to affect men as well as women.

A standard cure for women in older times with hysteria was scent therapy. It used good and bad scents to either compel the uterus one direction or the other or to chase the uterus back into place. For example if it is believed the woman's uterus is up by her mouth they would place the bad smell near her face to chase the uterus down. The good smell near her genitalia to lure the wandering uterus back down. This was a nice treatment. Ladies, does that sound pleasant to you?

It was also said that a woman's uterus was “sad and unfortunate" when it doesn't bear children or join with a male. This way of thinking played a role in the treatment for widowed and unmarried women to have sex or see a midwife for manual stimulation, using certain oils and scents to purge any fluid retention.

Some of the more harsh treatments included having the uterus removed if it was deemed uncontrollable. In some cases women were sent to asylums. We all know how well people were treated in asylums! French physician Philippe Pinel believed kindness and sensitivity were needed to create good care for these women.

The vibrator was originally designed to help with pain for many different diagnoses including arthritis, neuralgia, morbid irritability, indigestion, constipation, inflammation, tumors and more. Yes it was used in some cases to treat hysteria. And yes it did later become very well known for women's sexual pleasures.

It wasn't until the early 1900s that the idea of hysteria started to die off. How is it something we deem as merely being a part of being humans today was once a sin, demonic or problematic. Why is it that for so many centuries and even in parts of modern society women are still seen and treated as less than, weaker or of having more emotional problems? Is it really emotional problems or do women simply experience emotions differently than men? Anyone could go on for days asking similar questions.

Will science ever truly have all the answers? Or is part of human progress a constant cycle of questioning, testing, learning, and occasionally discovering that we were wrong?

For centuries, ideas about women, emotions, mental health, and the human body have shifted dramatically. Even today, debates continue over identity, biology, medicine, and how best to care for people experiencing distress. Some of today's most passionately defended beliefs may one day be reconsidered, just as countless beliefs before them were.

What ideas will society hold five years from now? Which of today's certainties will future generations question? And how many people will be affected before those answers become clear?

Moral Insanity

Moral Insanity is a term unfamiliar to most people today. During the 19th century it was a real diagnosis. Moral Insanity (Latin - mania sine delirio; French - folie raisonnante or folie lucide raisonnante, monomanie affective; German - Moralisches Irresein) was a medical diagnosis of mania without delusion. It was so prevalent that both moral insanity and monomania were depicted throughout Victorian novels and movies.

French psychiatrist Jean-Etienne Dominique Esquirol, a student of Philippe Pinel, developed the concept of monomania around 1810. It was a new diagnosis characterized by the presence of expansive fixed ideas, in which the mind was deranged or diseased in some areas but otherwise normal. There were three classifications of the mind, volitional, emotional and intellectual faculties. Emotional is when the patient is obsessed with one emotion or several related to it, intellectual is when it's only one kind of delirious idea or ideas. Volitional is a cognitive process by which an individual decides on and commits to a particular course of action.

Moral insanity was made possible due to the earlier works of two physicians. Philippe Pinel a French physician and zoologist working in Paris in 1778. He played an instrumental role in the development of a more humane psychological approach to the care and custody of psychiatric patients with a method referred to as moral therapy. Benjamin Rush an American physician who championed the idea of "partial madness" or that people could have varying degrees of mental illness. Rush was the first American to study mental disorders in a systematic manner. Rush died in 1813. More than a century later, in 1965, the American Psychiatric Association (APA) officially recognized him as the "Father of American Psychiatry."

In 1835 writing "Treatise on insanity and other disorders affecting the mind" James Cowles Prichard defined moral insanity as: "madness consisting in a morbid perversion of the natural feelings, affections, inclinations, temper, habits, moral dispositions, and natural impulses, without any remarkable disorder or defect of the interest or knowing and reasoning faculties, and particularly without any insane illusion or hallucinations." His theory was that moral insanity arose from a person's feelings and habits, not his intellect.

He believed there were four broad categories. Moral insanity, partial derangement, full mania, a breakdown of connections between ideas (incoherence or dementia). At the beginning of the 19th century views of insanity were just beginning to shift, from a view of demon possession which is untreatable, to a form of mental illness that was treatable. Moral treatment was referred to as a set of psychosocial techniques. Prichard used a mix of "moral treatments such as bleeding (bloodletting), vomiting and purging."

Alienists were physicians who specialized in mental disorders and would be called on to testify in courts and evaluate criminals. They were the 19th century version of what we in modern day consider a criminal/forensic psychologist. Alienists became the authoritative voice of psychiatry, they were responsible for the welfare of patients as well as the reputation of the institution. They were typically the Superintendents of the asylums.

The Association of Medical Superintendents of American Institutions for the Insane(AMSAII) or The Superintendents' Association, was created in October, 1844 in Philadelphia U.S.A.. A meeting of 13 superintendents from Massachusetts, Maine, Rhode Island, Connecticut, New York, Philadelphia, Pennsylvania, Ohio and Virginia. It was known as the first professional Medical specialty organization in the U.S.A. . The objective of the AMSAII was "to communicate their experiences to each other, cooperate in collecting statistical information relating to insanity, and assist each other in improving the treatment of the insane." In 1921, AMSAII officially became the American Psychiatric Association (APA).

When it came to involuntary commitment of alleged insane individuals, Prichard was cautious in using the diagnosis. His typical clients tended to be the educated class who held asylums in low regard. "Of all these arrangements the maintenance of public order is the principal object, and the second is the preservation of the property belonging to the lunatic and the interest of his family."

Though Prichard developed the concept of moral insanity with the intention of improving the treatment of mental illness, the diagnosis gradually became a tool of social control. Behaviors that challenged social expectations could increasingly be interpreted as evidence of disorder rather than individuality. A woman who mourned longer than the community considered appropriate, she must have a disorder. A daughter rejected the arranged marriage because she was mentally unbalanced. A woman who cried after giving birth was morally unstable. The frequency at which interpretations like those grew as time progressed. With a heavy target towards women who didn't conform.

What we consider feelings now was a diagnosis of moral insanity in the 19th century. Those beliefs led to some bizarre medical records and also led to the confinement and abuse of countless women. Once a woman was given the diagnosis it became difficult for her to protest as her attempts would be seen as proof of the diagnosis.

The true power behind moral insanity was how easily it fit into the social and legal structures of the time. 19th century families were hierarchies where husbands held authority over their households. Community leaders decided and set the moral tone while fathers made decisions for the household. When a woman did anything that stepped outside those boundaries "moral insanity" offered people an explanation that still preserved the hierarchy.

A few physicians warned that families were using the asylum system to get rid of inconvenient relatives. Newspapers occasionally commented on the growing number of women in confinement for reasons that had nothing to do with madness. It still stuck due to how neatly it fit into the boarder beliefs. Women were expected to be dependent, agreeable, and quiet anything beyond that could get women labeled as morally insane.

A woman in the asylum who showed any emotion was often seen as further proof that she was unstable or insane. Women were monitored for emotions, they were put on strict schedules to exclude individuality. Some asylums relied heavily on physical restraint while others used isolation rooms. Women who went in sane wound up deteriorating under those conditions creating the appearance of illness where there were none.

Would you really want to live back then? Would you survive the asylum or increasingly absurd diagnoses that sent people to asylums? Would you have been diagnosed with moral insanity?

Witch Trials/Witch Hunts

A lot of people here in the U.S.A. think that the Salem Witch Trials were bad. There is a lot of lore surrounding it, it is a part of almost every Halloween in some way. Witches! Beware the satanic witches! A warning that has been echoed throughout time. For those who believe in the Bible, the earliest biblical references to witches are dated 900-700 BC. For those of you who prefer historical dating, witches were documented in ancient Greece and Rome. The belief in witches has changed as time has progressed. In earlier times witches were seen as evil and something that must be stopped. So much so that there were laws written against doing supernatural harm.

Witchcraft and the belief in it has led to many tragic events throughout history. Looking back it is hard for people to accurately say how many people have suffered/lost their lives for being believed to be witches or possessing supernatural abilities. Some of the more infamous witch trials were the Europe Witch Trials from 1400-1775 and the Salem Witch Trials in the USA starting in 1692 and ending in 1693. Trials took place in France, Germany, Austria, United States of America, Switzerland and parts of the UK. Oddly, the Salem Witch Trials receive far more attention in books, movies, and popular culture than the much larger European witch trials.

The world had just begun to recover from the Black Death (the Black Plague). If you aren't familiar with the Black Death, go look it up. The witch trials' final years were the beginning years of the Industrial Revolution. The Hundred Years' War between France and England ended in 1453 just a few decades after the trials began. 1492 Columbus sailed the ocean blue, how many times have you heard that? 1492 America saw the first tiny starts of our nation, as the European witch trials were reaching their first century. One year after the Witch Trials of Europe ended, America gained its Independence. It's truly astounding how many things changed while the European Witch Hunts ravaged the lands.

The European trials were more akin to witch hunts. They lasted centuries whereas the Salem Witch Trials only lasted one year. The witch trials in Europe saw between 40,000-60,000 executions, mostly women. The majority of the deaths occurred during "the Great Hunt" (peak 1560-1630). Driven by social tensions, religious turmoil, and the fear of a "Devil's pact". They believed witches sometimes took flight to go to witches sabbaths, a nocturnal gathering where Witches worshiped Demons and Satan, where they engaged in cannibalism, sexual orgies and infanticide. Those people in return would gain supernatural powers from the devil.

Legal procedures ("inquisitorial" procedures), involving accusations based on outlandish rumors and "the swimming test" torture, were used to gain names of accomplices and confessions. If a woman was found guilty of being a witch, which she usually was, the punishments ranged. Punishment often led to burning them at the stake (at times alive, others strangled first), hanging, life imprisonment, banishment/Exile, decapitation, strangulation, ducking stool, public humiliation depending on where you lived and how severe the "case" against you was.

Most of the women who lost their lives were not witches. It was very common for someone to make accusations against someone who cared for another who died, it was blamed on the caretaker. A midwife helps deliver a baby and the baby dies; suddenly she is accused of being a witch. People who were accused usually faced torture to extract a "confession". Women if you were alive in this time would you be so inclined to help others? Would you make that herbal tea you love so much?

Often the "Witches" who were accused never made it to trial, they died during torture or in prison. In several countries men were accused as well as women such as Finland, Estonia, Iceland and Russia. It really came down to where you lived and what the beliefs of those in the society around you held. The Salem Witch Trials were prominent when the European trials died off. The end of the trials was the late 17th to 18th century, the last often unofficial executions occurring in places like Switzerland in 1782 and Poland in 1793.

Germany is known for some of the largest documented witch trials in history, resulting in thousands of executions across multiple regions. The Trier witch trials, Fulda witch trials, Würzburg witch trials, and Bamberg witch trials formed the four largest witch trials in Germany. The Witch Trials of Trier took place in the diocese of Trier in the Holy Roman Empire (present day Germany) between 1581-1593. The trials started in the diocese of Trier in 1581 only making its way to the city in 1587. The city itself saw 368 people executed in only five years, making it potentially one of the largest mass executions in Europe in a time of peace.

The Würzburg witch trials of 1625-1631 which took place in the self-governing Catholic Prince-Bishopric of Würzburg in the Holy Roman Empire. In a land where ongoing religious Thirty Years War between the Catholics and Protestants. In an area on the border between Protestant and Catholic territories. 219 are estimated to have been executed in the city, while another 900 were executed or died in the custody of Prince-Bishopric.

The Bamberg witch trials of 1627-1632 which also took place in the self-governing Catholic Prince-Bishopric of Bamberg in the Holy Roman Empire. During those short five years around 1,000 people were executed for witchcraft. Yet another territory that was riddled with witch trials caught between a religious/power war.

Witch trials throughout the world left a trail of fear, suspicion, and bloodshed that lasted for centuries. Communities became convinced that hidden enemies were responsible for their suffering, and once those fears took hold, evidence often became secondary to belief.

For centuries humanity has feared the unknown. Sometimes that fear created caution. Other times it created victims.

What will be the next witch hunt? Will it ever truly end?

SATANIC PANIC 1980'S-1990'S

Satanic Panic originated in 1980 with the release/publication of a book called Michelle Remembers. The book was co-written by Canadian psychiatrist Lawrence Pazder and his patient/future wife Michelle Smith. The book used the now discredited and controversial practice of Recovered Memory Therapy (RMT) to make claims about Satanic ritual abuse involving Michelle.

The book claims all of this happened when Michelle was five years old and that the memories were later recovered during sessions with Lawrence. The book made claims of an 81 day ritual involving the summoning of Satan with Jesus, the Virgin Mary and Michael the Archangel intervening and healing all of her wounds while blocking her memories of it. The book claims Michelle was locked in cages, forced to participate in various rituals, tortured, sexually assaulted, witnessed several human sacrifices, and had the body parts and blood of sacrificed adults and infants. The book claims all of this happened to Michelle when she was 5 years old and the memories were recovered through her sessions with Lawrence. The book was a chronicle of their sessions.

Even though every allegation/claim made in the book was debunked there was still a massive following of people who fully believed it. Allegations of both sexual and physical abuse in the context of Satanic or Occult rituals spread rapidly across the U.S.A. . Some allegations ring eerily similar to the modern day theories about a group of hidden elite who abduct children and breed them for human sacrifice, pornography, prostitution and run a global Satanic cult. Many believed the panic ended in the 1990s... but similar patterns of moral panic and accusations of hidden elite abuse continue to surface today. How much has really changed?

The panic affected not only the public but it also affected a lot of lawyers, social workers, religious fundamentalists, police investigators, therapists, clients in psychotherapy and the media. Lawrence and Michelle toured the U.S.A. promoting "Michelle Remembers" they became celebrities, Oprah Winfrey had Michelle on her show 10 years after the book was published. Everywhere their book was being pushed as fact. It was referenced at police seminars, psychology conventions and court cases.

Testimonials, rumors, symptom lists and techniques to investigate / uncover satanic ritual abuse were talked about and passed around on talk shows, professional circles, religious groups, and conferences. This not only prolonged the panic but helped spread it beyond the United States. Over 12,000 unsubstantiated cases of SRA Satanic Ritual Abuse were made in just over 10 years.

Michelle's own family spoke out against her claims. People did research, publishing stories about how her timelines don't add up to the facts of her actual life. One example is the 81 day long ritual, she claims to have happened, researchers found she was still showing up to school unharmed. Yet her claims are that she was tortured. She claims the abuse happened because of her mother, yet not once were her two sisters mentioned.

In 1994 Pat Pulling joined with psychiatrist Tomas Radecki to create B.A.D.D (Bothered About Dungeons and Dragons). Yes, that really was the name of it! They claimed general role play games, especially Dungeons and Dragons, were recruitment tools for Satanism. They alleged the games caused the young to murder, Satanic ritual abuse and commit suicide. They also pointed to heavy metal music, educators, childcare centers, and television. Ironically studies from that time frame actually found that kids who played role play games were less likely to be suicidal.

The SRA panic echoes many dark chapters throughout history all the way back from 16th and 17th century witch hunts to modern day. It even appears in the bible (Genesis 3:13- "The serpent deceived me, and I ate"- the classic "the devil made me do it"). How many times have we heard that excuse? How many times have we blamed games/heavy metal music for society's problems? How much do we really know or understand about what happened then... or even now?

Want to Dig Deeper?

The following pages contain links to museum collections, archives, historical photographs, public records, documentaries, and other resources related to each section of this book.

Scan the QR code or type the web address to continue your investigation.

MASS HYSTERIA / FEMALE HYSTERIA

Explore:

https://www.historic-uk.com/CultureUK/Hysterical-Victorian-Women/

THE WITCH TRIALS / WITCH HUNTS

Explore:

https://www.youtube.com/watch?v=r9TzCoEGyr4

THE SATANIC PANIC (1980S–1990S)

Explore:

https://www.youtube.com/watch?v=plEImKEIRm8

Part III

Medical Denial & Harm

RECOVERED MEMORY THEORY

Recovered Memory Therapy (RMT) was used to help people "recall" supposedly forgotten memories, especially traumatic ones from childhood. Some therapists and patients believed in it wholeheartedly. Others have spent decades trying to discredit it. In the 1980s and 1990s, the practice exploded. Therapists used techniques like hypnosis, age regression, guided visualization, repeated interviews, and sometimes the drug Sodium Amytal (Often called a "truth serum") to supposedly unlock repressed memories. If you aren't sure what Sodium Amytal is, I would highly recommend you look up Sodium Amytal before moving on to the next section.

One 2018 study found that about 5% of participants reported recovering memories of abuse they had no previous recollection of. However, research by psychologist Elizabeth Loftus and others showed how dangerously easy it is to create entirely false memories. They used methods like the "familial informant false narrative procedure" — essentially telling someone a family member had confirmed an event happened, then reinforcing it through suggestion and repeated "memory exercises." The human cost was significant.

Patients sometimes became absolutely convinced of horrific events that never actually occurred. Many walked away with absolute conviction that the false memory was real. This led to psychological distress, broken family relationships, wrongful accusations, increased anxiety, fear, and depression. The ripple effects destroyed families and reputations. How many lives were upended because a therapist was certain they were helping someone "remember"? How do we know today which memories are genuine and which were planted? And perhaps most uncomfortable: what techniques are we still using in therapy or self-help circles that future generations might look back on with the same questioning?

Ignaz Semmelweis & Handwashing 1840s–1860s

Ignaz was bothered by the difference in death rates from puerpenal fever of two clinics. He began trying to figure out what was causing a higher rate of death in one of the clinics. He tried putting women in different positions during birth, even proposed the idea that the priests that were coming in were terrifying them and causing the fever. It wasn't until his colleague, Jakob Kolletschka died after his hand was cut during an autopsy of someone who died of childbed fever. The pathology report showed something similar to puerperal fever. He proposed the idea that students and doctors carried "cadaverous particles" on their hands and they were causing the problems.

Ignaz started experimenting on himself, trying several methods to wash his hands. Chlorinated lime is what he found worked best to remove the odor of infected autopsy tissue, he thought perhaps it would destroy any "cadaveric particles". Chlorinated lime was also used to sterilize drinking water, whiten paper and clean stables. He put in a policy for washing hands between autopsies and examination of patients. After implementing the new policy in April of 1847 the clinic saw a progressing decrease in mortality rate. Before it was implemented the mortality rate was 18.3% by August it had dropped to 1.9%. It took a matter of months before his technique almost completely wiped out the fever.

During 1848 he widened his scope of washing to include all instruments that came in contact with patients. His idea began to expand to include the concept that all decaying organic matter was a potential risk. By 1849, Ignaz was obliged to leave his clinic. After leaving, he worked as a docent (a private lecturer who taught students) in 1850. They had refused him access to cadavers, limiting his teaching to mannequins only. Due to this only a few days after being notified of his appointment for docent he left for Pest.

In Pest, Ignaz took the position of head-physician of obstetrics of Szent Rókus on May 20th, 1851. Childbed fever was rampant at the clinic when he visited in 1850. During 1851-1855 Ignaz virtually eliminated the disease with only eight patients dying out of 933 births. Despite his results his ideas were not accepted by other obstetricians in Budapest. He wrote a book about his work, Die Ätiologie, der Begriff und die Prophylaxis des Kindbettfiebers (German for "The Etiology, Concept and Prophylaxis of Childbed Fever") in 1861.

Ignaz sent copies of his book to scientific institutions and prominent obstetricians across Europe. He had hoped that by sending his book with his findings it would change the understanding of Childbed Fever. His idea conflicted with the established opinions at the time. It was believed that diseases were due to an imbalance in the "four humours". They believed each case was uniquely precise to the patient so it couldn't be widespread. Due to the beliefs at the time Ignaz's theory was dismissed by most of the medical field. Some doctors were offended at the idea that their hands were unclean. The widespread rejection affected him heavily.

In his frustrations over the rejections Ignaz wrote letters addressed to the International Medical Community. He expressed his disappointment and anger at the "massacre" he believed his fellow colleagues were responsible for. "It weighs on my conscience that thousands upon thousands of mothers and infants have perished—lives that could have been saved...The killing must end, and to bring it to an end I shall stand guard. Whoever dares to promote dangerous doctrines about childbed fever will find in me a resolute opponent."

Over time, his psychological state deteriorated. In 1865 János Balassa wrote a document referring Ignaz to a mental institution. He was lured by Ferdinand Ritter von Hebra under the pretense of visiting one of Hebra's "new institutes". Ignaz caught on to what was happening and tried to escape but was caught severely beaten and secured in a straitjacket then confined in a dark cell. Some of the "treatments" Ignaz endured were dousing with cold water, giving him castor oil and a laxative. After only two weeks on August 13th, 1865 Ignaz died of a gangrenous wound.

Over time, his psychological state deteriorated. In 1865 János Balassa wrote a document referring Ignaz to a mental institution. He was lured by Ferdinand Ritter von Hebra under the pretense of visiting one of Hebra's "new institutes". Ignaz caught on to what was happening and tried to escape but was caught severely beaten and secured in a straitjacket then confined in a dark cell. Some of the "treatments" Ignaz endured were dousing with cold water, giving him castor oil and a laxative. After only two weeks on August 13th, 1865 Ignaz died of a gangrenous wound.

It was in 1861 that Louis Pasteur published a paper formally presenting his germ theory. By 1864, Louis had begun public experiments. As Ignaz sat dying in an asylum, Pasteur was producing evidence that supported what Ignaz had been arguing for years. He died in that same institution in 1865. It was only after Ignaz's death that his findings were accepted due to germ theory. Notice a trend in our history? How many people only get recognition after they are dead and treated as crazy when they are alive? How many "crazy" ideas will be the norm in the next decade?

Smoking Advertised as Healthy 1920s–1960s

Doctor recommended brand! As your Dentist I would recommend this brand. When have you heard that in regards to cigarettes? To think, three generations ago it was promoted as healthy even for the young and pregnant women. It was pushed as an appetite suppression to keep you thin, as a way to make you look "cool", good for digestion, anxiety issues, to help you feel your best etc. Completely absurd by today's standards, yet completely accepted at the time.

R.J. Reynolds Tobacco Company created a Medical Relations Division. They began paying for research and citing the data in ads. One of those ad campaigns was "More doctors smoke Camels than any other cigarette." They would give doctors a free carton of Camels then ask them what brand they liked and boom doctor recommended.

Many companies used celebrities to advertise for their brand. They used pictures of elites smoking their brand while at "parties". Tobacco companies even used landmarks to advertise their brand. Everywhere you turned, smoking was being promoted as healthy. Not just by the tobacco companies but it was being pushed by doctors. Tobacco ads on television and radio were banned in 1971 due to the growing concerns about damages.

By 1964 the U.S. Surgeon General's report came out that stated, smoking caused lung cancer, laryngeal cancer, and chronic bronchitis. American Tobacco Company funded "research" that downplayed risks. They claimed there was still a "controversy" over whether cigarettes were unhealthy until 1998. Millions lost their lives, and millions more continue to suffer the consequences today. Why have we not learned our lesson? What are we being told now that is good for us is actually toxic? I'm sure many examples come to mind, especially when looking at today's processed food industry.

RADIUM GIRLS 1910S–1920S

Radium was identified by Pierre and Marie Curie in 1898 and successfully isolated a few years after. The couple knew it was dangerous, both had burns and felt the effects of radiation sickness. They found it could destroy "sick cells", in doing so radium soon became seen as a cure to anything and everything. It was put in cosmetics, chocolate, tonic water, toothpaste and eventually into beer and bread.

Due to Industrialization, economic necessity and labor shortages caused by World War I (WWI), the amount of women joining the work force increased. Before this time period women were seen as the ones to stay at home while the man worked. One of these new factory roles for women was to paint glow-in-the-dark watch dials as well as military instruments. The girls who worked at the watch factories were told it was safe and encouraged to lick the brushes to make it easier to paint the detail work on watches and dials. This was a highly sought after job as it was easy light work and paid up to three times more than other jobs.

Radium is a naturally occurring, highly radioactive, silvery-white metal known for its luminescent effect. Most of you probably already have thoughts that come to mind when you hear the word "radioactive." Radium dust got all over the women's hair, skin, and clothes as they worked, giving them a sparkle and glow. Some of the women started wearing their finest dresses to work so they could glow while dancing on the weekends. A few of the women applied it to their teeth to "give their kiss a pop". These women got the name of "Radium Girls" or the more widely known "Ghost Girls".

The women exposed to the radium had toothaches, bleeding gums, severe anemia, mouth sores, painful gums and jaws, exhaustion, blood cancer, leukemia infections, loss of teeth, struggling to eat due to pain, it can cause you to become sterile, Radium Jaw (jaw necrosis) sometimes leading to the removal of the lower jaw, bone tumors, and eventually death.

These women were made to believe it was safe, told they were beautiful because of the glow effect and they believed it so much it eventually killed them. How much is beauty worth to you ladies?

One of the Radium Girls, Mollie Maggia in January of 1922 went to her dentist for a toothache. The dentist pulled the tooth and another tooth, he noticed her wounds didn't heal. Mollie eventually had to have surgery on a fast growing abscess that was growing on her jaw. During the surgery the dentist noticed her jaw looked gray and ashy. After gently poking at it her jaw crumbled under his touch leading to the removal of the remaining parts of her jaw in the following summer. Mollie died just before her 25th birthday; her death was listed as syphilis. She had developed tumors in her throat that cut into her jugular vein causing her to choke to death on her blood.

In the early 1920s, the United States Radium Corporation contacted Harvard School of Public Health researchers Cecil Kent Drinker and his wife, Katherine Rotan Drinker. The Drinkers were to examine the Orange, New Jersey factory and determine why several employees had fallen "ill". Drinker thought the employees constant heavy exposure to radium was causing the health problems the employees were having. Watch dial companies rejected the claims that workers were suffering from radium exposure.

Women were often told it was the X-ray that caused the radiation problems. Under pressure from the dial company, medical professionals listed workers' deaths as things like syphilis. They also made claims that they hired "a great many people who were physically unfit to procure employment in other lines of industry" out of kindness. Arthur Roeder, the president of the company threatened to sue Drinker if he published his findings. Drinker published it anyway, inadvertently starting lawsuits as well as permanent changes in the factory industry.

By 1923, one of the radium girls who had already had her jaw fall away from her skull, died. By 1924, 50 women fell ill and a dozen were dead. Grace Fryer spent two years looking for an attorney willing to take on the USRC. By the time the five women who were in the lawsuit saw their first court appearance in January of 1928 two were bedridden and none were capable of raising their arms to take the oath. Grace Fryer, Edna Hussman, Katherine Schaub, Albania Larice and Quinta McDonald are the five women more infamously known as The Radium Girls from this court case.

The turning point for these women was 1927-1928 where lawsuits and media exposure helped draw attention to what had happened. The case was settled in autumn 1928 before it ever reached a jury, USRC (U.S. Radium Corporation) denied any wrongdoing. A cash settlement was awarded to the girls as well as all medical and legal expenses would be paid by the company. Mind you this is only for the New Jersey women. The New Jersey women died by the 1930s.

In Illinois employees began asking for compensation for medical and dental bills in 1927. The first lawsuit brought before the Illinois Industrial Commission (IIC) was in 1937. In spring of 1938 the IIC ruled in favor of the women, but the company Radium Dial had closed and moved to New York. Radium Dial appealed to the U.S Supreme Court and on October 23rd, 1939 the court decided not to hear the appeal and the lower court's ruling was upheld. Some of the women never received any payout and one of the 5 women was dead by time the court case was fully settled.

The Radium Girls and these court cases helped to establish workers compensation laws and radiation safety standards. In 1949 Congress passed a bill that granted compensation for all workers suffering from occupational diseases. Radium Dial painters were given safety precautions, stopped shaping the brush with their lips, and provided protective gear. The data measurements from 27 dial painters was used in 1941 by the National Bureau of Standards to establish a tolerance for radium.

So the next time you see a radioactive warning symbol and understand the dangers it represents, remember the women whose suffering helped establish the safety standards and protections that exist today.

What products, treatments, or technologies do we use every day because we believe they are safe? Which of them will future generations discover carried risks we failed to recognize? How many are already on that list?

Transorbital Lobotomy of Walter Freeman II 1930s–1960s

Walter Freeman II was an American neurologist who wanted to simplify lobotomies. Psychiatric hospitals often did not have access to operating rooms, anesthesia surgeons, and limited budgets. As Freeman was only a neurologist and not a neurosurgeon he enlisted the help of neurosurgeon James Watts. When they first started out they were performing what Freeman named the lobotomy.

A prefrontal lobotomy was a modified leucotomy, instead of drilling holes in the frontal lobe like with leucotomy the prefrontal lobotomy severed the connections to and from the prefrontal cortex. Due to the fact that these procedures required drilling into the patients head they had to be performed in an operating room by trained neurosurgeons.

Freeman popularized a transorbital lobotomy procedure. The procedure involved using an orbitoclast (an instrument that resembles an ice pick) under the eyelid and against the top of the eye socket; a mallet was then used to drive the “ice pick” through the thin layer of bone into the prefrontal cortex. After the orbitoclast was inserted it was swept laterally to obliterate the frontal lobe tissue. This new procedure was used without anesthesia instead using electroconvulsive therapy to induce seizure. The portable electroshock machines enabled doctors to perform this procedure in an office setting.

In 1947 Watts left due to his opposition to the transorbital lobotomy. Freeman began traveling across the country visiting institutions performing lobotomies and spreading his views/ methods. Most of these operations were performed for free as demonstrations.

Symptoms that required a lobotomy were anxiety, OCD, depression, psychosis, schizophrenia, even "difficult" behavior. Usually done in asylums where treatments ranged from, malarial therapy for general paresis of the insane, cardiazol shock therapy, deep sleep therapy, insulin shock therapy, electroconvulsive therapy and lobotomies.

Over 40,000-50,000 lobotomies were performed in the U.S.A. alone. 25-30 years and over 40,000 people were forever changed by "surgically induced childhood". A term Walter coined himself to describe the state that patients were after lobotomies.

The operation left people with severe personality changes, cognitive impairment, or they became vegetables, decreased cognition, detachment from society, incontinence, some gained enormous appetites leading to considerable weight gain, brain abscess, intracranial hemorrhage, epilepsy, dementia, and even death.

Key functions were dramatically reduced after the procedure such as, responsiveness, spontaneity, and self-awareness.

Freeman described a 29 year old woman as being a "smiling, lazy and satisfactory patient with the personality of an oyster" after a lobotomy. She couldn't remember his name and just kept pouring an empty pot of coffee. When her parents struggled to deal with this new her they were recommended to do a system of rewards (ice cream) and punishments (smacks).

One of the more famous patients of Freeman was Rosemary Kennedy, sister of President John F. Kennedy. Due to a Spanish influenza epidemic and no doctors available the nurse forced the baby to stay in the birth canal for two hours. The actions of the staff resulted in a loss of oxygen which caused delays in Rosemary's basic developmental steps. In 1941 at the age of 23 Rosemary became increasingly irritable and difficult as well as declining in concentration, memory and judgement. After doctors convinced her father that a lobotomy would help calm her mood swings and stop her occasional violent outbursts, he arranged for her to have a lobotomy without her mothers knowledge

After Freeman had already performed five thousand lobotomies his methods were questioned for being unreliable and unethical. By 1954 the invention of drugs such as chlorpromazine offered patients and families safer alternatives to lobotomies. The risks and consequences of lobotomies and the fact lobotomies were no longer profitable caused physicians to start using chlorpromazine and other prescription drugs.

This was common practice back then. Would you let a doctor give someone you loved a lobotomy if you were convinced it would help? Lobotomies were a common treatment in asylums. It permanently changed peoples lives ruining them more often then not. I would recommend reading The Lobotomy Patient—A Decade Later A Follow-up Study of a Research Project Started in 1948. The study noted that 91% of patients exhibited a "Personality Defect", which typically diminished spontaneity, self-control, creativity, responsiveness, and leading to apathy or emotional flattening. This study was conducted prior to the adoption of antipsychotic drugs like Chlorpromazine ruling lobotomies obsolete.

Curious Atrocities Part III

Mental Disorders/Asylums and Treatments

In old times, mental disorders were thought to have been caused by supernatural forces such as demons or spirits. This belief led to a lot of inhumane treatments, including incarceration in dungeons. Have you seen/heard of the way people who were put in dungeons were treated, if not I would recommend looking into it. During the "Dark ages" the heavy beliefs in folk lore, theology, and the occult, people who were deemed "Mad" were often treated terribly.

In the 19th and 20th centuries mad houses became lunatic asylums. Treatments in this era ranged from straight jackets, electroshock therapy, insulin injections, cold or hot treatments, lobotomies, chaining patients to beds, chairs, or walls and worse. The lunatic/insane asylums have long since been a part of the halloween lore for their creepy vibes, due to the horrific treatment the patients endured.

A notable example of asylums gone wrong is Crownsville State Hospital Maryland. In 1953 there was an uprising. Tear gas and fire hoses were used against patients rioting for better conditions. There are photos of firemen spraying a burning mattress that was thrown from a window by patients. Guards locked themselves in the bathrooms. It was a 556 acre farm where patients helped build many of the structures on the grounds, milked cows, harvested willow for making furniture and baskets, and tended crops.

Patients included homeless kids, people with syphilis, the criminally insane, the mentally ill, drunks, and people with tuberculosis. Mortality rates were tragically high – It's estimated that about 1,800 patients were buried there, with approximately 1,400 unnamed, numbered graves. The ledger that would have identified many of them has been lost or destroyed.

The 1950s riots were blamed on operating the facility both as a mental hospital and a penal institution. Overcrowding made the blend “nessacary”. Originally, it was an institution where only Negroes were due to their beliefs at the time that they needed to be kept separate from whites; it was later integrated. It wasn't unheard of for staff to use patients as test subjects for new treatment methods, sometimes portrayed as a way for patients to “pay back” the institution for being there.

One of the pioneers for a more humane approach was Philippe Pinel. He became chief physician at the Paris asylum Bicêtre, an asylum for men. He made the then bold choice to unchain the patients, many who had been chained for up to 30 or 40 years. He later did the same for the inmates of Salpêtrière where he became director in 1794. He took an approach that later became known as talk therapy, where he would talk to the patients about their problems.

Mental illness throughout history has been viewed as supernatural, biological, psychological problems. Our understanding of it has grown and evolved with time. How much will our understanding change in say 30 years? What will all be changed? How much of what we really think we know today could we be wrong about? Anywhere you look in regards to asylums/sanatoriums etc. you will find similar horror stories on how the patients were treated. I could go on for weeks talking about the many different ones and the things that happened in them. I will instead simply suggest that you yourself look into it if you haven't already.

Want to Dig Deeper?

The following pages contain links to museum collections, archives, historical photographs, public records, documentaries, and other resources related to each section of this book.

Scan the QR code or type the web address to continue your investigation.

Ignaz Semmelweis and the Fight for Handwashing

Explore:

https://www.sciencehistory.org/education/scientific-biographies/ignaz-semmelweis/

Smoking Advertised as Healthy

Explore:

https://rarehistoricalphotos.com/bizarre-vintage-tobacco-advertising/

The Radium Girls

Explore:

https://www.kate-moore.com/the-radium-girls

Transorbital Lobotomy of Walter Freeman II

Explore:

https://pmc.ncbi.nlm.nih.gov/articles/PMC1922743/

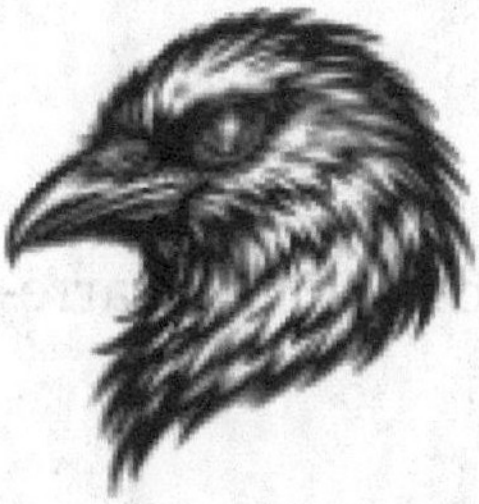

PART IV

STATE POWER, GOVERNMENT ABUSE & COVER UPS

Drapetomania

Samuel A. Cartwright proposed the mental illness of Drapetomania in 1851. His hypothesis was based on a belief that slavery was such an improvement of the lives of slaves that only those suffering from some form of mental illness would be willing to escape. His theory was Drapetomania the reason enslaved Americans fled captivity was a mental illness. It sounds absurd today, but to many people at the time it seemed perfectly reasonable.

Mostly reprinted in the South, his article was widely satirized and mocked in the northern United States. He is quoted saying "If treated kindly, well fed and clothed, with fuel enough to keep a small fire burning all night—separated into families, each family having its own house—not permitted to run about at night to visit their neighbors, to receive visits or use intoxicating liquors, and not overworked or exposed too much to the weather, they are very easily governed—more so than any other people in the world. If any one or more of them, at any time, are inclined to raise their heads to a level with their master or overseer, humanity and their own good requires that they should be punished until they fall into that submissive state which was intended for them to occupy. They have only to be kept in that state, and treated like children to prevent and cure them from running away."

He even tried to use the Bible to push his beliefs. "If the white man attempts to oppose the Deity's will, by trying to make the negro anything else than "the submissive knee-bender" (which the Almighty declared he should be), by trying to raise him to a level with himself, or by putting himself on an equality with the negro; or if he abuses the power which God has given him over his fellow-man, by being cruel to him, or punishing him in anger, or by neglecting to protect him from the wanton abuses of his fellow-servants and all others, or by denying him the usual comforts and necessaries of life, the negro will run away; but if he keeps him in the position that we learn from the Scriptures he was intended to occupy, that is, the position of submission; and if his master or overseer be kind and gracious in his bearing towards him, without condescension, and at the same time ministers to his physical wants, and protects him from abuses, the negro is spell-bound, and cannot run away."

How did he manage to frame such blatant racism and control as kindness and good treatment? At the same time he encouraged that if you thought your slave was being sulky or dissatisfied without cause you should whip the devil out of them as a preventive measure. His works were mocked so much in the north, Frederick Law Olmsted wrote A Journey in the Seaboard Slave States in 1856. Frederick observed that white indentured servants had often been known to flee as well, so he satirically hypothesized that the supposed disease was actually of white European origin, and had been introduced to Africa by traders. Even with the scrutiny and mockery, parts of the South continued to embrace the theory. How many more generations will people continue dividing one another into categories of "us" and "them"? Will race remain the dividing line, or will something else take its place? Will you be a part of the next divide? Will it be something other than race?

Sluggish Schizophrenia

Schizophrenia is still a recognized mental illness that can negatively affect a person's quality of life. Early diagnosis and treatment are essential for people. A Soviet psychiatrist named Andrei Snezhnevsky developed the diagnostic criteria for sluggish schizophrenia. It was used by psychiatrists and doctors in the USSR and some eastern block countries until 1989 when the fall of communism began.

Psychiatry became a method of control over one's mental state. This diagnosis was widely regarded as a tool for political control rather than genuine medical treatment. Sluggish schizophrenia was a mental health diagnosis. It was used by the Soviet Union during the post World War II era. People could receive a diagnosis with no symptoms of schizophrenia or psychosis. Doctors claimed that symptoms could appear at any time.

The Institute of Psychiatry of the Academy of Medical Sciences of the USSR defined three forms of schizophrenia, depending on whether the condition was continuous, recurrent or mixed. There were three subtypes that people would fall into.

Pseudoneurotic Form (Anxiety-like)- This subtype presents symptoms similar to obsessive-compulsive disorder, neuroses, or hypochondria. Patients experienced intense unexplainable phobias, anxiety or constant focus with bodily discomfort.

Pseudopsychopathic Form (Behavioral nonconformity)- This subtype is characterized by noticeable changes in behavior, personality, and emotion. Patients may exhibit loss of drive, eccentric habits, emotional blunting, eccentric behaviors that can be misinterpreted as a personality disorder, and a drop in productivity.

Paranoid Form (Overvalued ideas)- a slow development of "overvalued ideas" or singular obsessions. Patients may become intensely focused on a specific philosophical, intellectual, or reformist pursuit. Often leading to neglect of all other areas of their life.

Many experts believe that Snezhnevsky developed the diagnosis of sluggish schizophrenia due to requests from the Communist Party. The underlying logic was that anyone who opposed the Soviet regime must be mentally ill, because no rational person would reject the system. Diagnosing individuals with sluggish schizophrenia became a tool for handling political dissent.

Individuals who were involved in publication or distribution of anti-state literature or political activists were targets. Psychiatrists would incarcerate these people into mental asylums without any justification. Under the Soviet era laws these people could be placed in maximum security hospitals and or prison camps.

"Admitting" to one's incorrect behaviors was often not enough to overturn a diagnosis. To ensure the reeducation was successful, sane dissidents who recanted their previous objections against the government would be held for years in isolation. Historian Robert van Voren explained, lower-ranking psychiatric institutions such as regional outpatient clinics never dared overturn a diagnosis made by a large psychiatric hospital. Thus enabling these patients/dissidents to remain locked up for years. The thinking at the time was that asylums provided a place where "unreason" could be isolated, contained, and prevented from influencing others. This was happening throughout the world, not just in Russia.

GULF WAR SYNDROME 1990S–PRESENT

This is a tricky subject. Veterans in America are honored, loved and respected by many. They sacrifice so much so we can live our lives with the freedoms we were granted back in 1776 and everything since. For hundreds of years men have fought and died for not only our freedoms but for others freedoms as well. They have fought to protect those who can't. Because of that they have not always been treated with the respect they deserve by our own government.

The United States joined the Persian Gulf War in 1990 due to a combination of compelling threats. Iraq's annexation of Kuwait gave Saddam Hussein control over around 20% of the world's oil reserves. President George H.W. Bush led Operation Desert Storm, to prevent hostile powers from dominating the Middle East and to ensure the protection of the flow of oil.

Soldiers returned with a slew of unexplained chronic symptoms that include fatigue, headaches, joint pain, indigestion, cognitive problems, diarrhea, insomnia, muscle pain, dizziness, respiratory disorders, and memory problems. Granted they didn't all get hit with all of those symptoms. Imagine getting hit with one or two or even three of those while dealing with readjusting to "normal" life again. The diagnosis for these men was Undiagnosed illness, chronic multisymptom illness and later Gulf War illness.

It is a heavily debated theory that Gulf War Syndrome could be a post-infectious problem linked to exposure to sub-lethal amounts of cyclosarin and sarin — organophosphate nerve agents released atmospherically during the war. Researchers have investigated several possible contributing factors, including exposure to sarin and cyclosarin nerve agents, pesticides, oil well fire smoke, and pyridostigmine bromide (PB) tablets that were issued as a protective measure against nerve-agent exposure.

While evidence suggests some of these exposures may have played a role, the exact causes of Gulf War Illness remain a subject of ongoing research. Approximately 30-40% of those who served have chronic multi-symptom illness. This is an approximation the numbers are still under debate and changing.

In 2017 GAO (Government Accountability Office) published a report stating the VA denied the majority of Gulf War illness claims. It was also found that the denial rates were higher than for all other medical issues related to war. The claims process was longer for those submitting Gulf War illness claims. It is still debated to this day though the VA recognizes some symptoms as service related. There are veterans who put themselves on the line for the U.S.A to come home sometimes in chronic pain, struggling to adjust, or haunted by the things they endured. Only to be fighting for help to control the storm within themselves, against the very people they fought for. Think about that one long and hard next time you see that military patch on that old man's arm or hat.

History shows that governments are often eager to send men and women into harm's way, but not always as eager to care for them when they return home. Gulf War Syndrome is only one example among many where veterans spent years fighting to have their suffering acknowledged. For some, the war did not end when they came home—it simply changed forms. This mistreatment of our soldiers is a topic that just never seems to go away, no matter how many centuries pass.

TUSKEGEE SYPHILIS EXPERIMENTS 1932-1972

In 1932 the U.S. Public Health Service working with Tuskegee Institute began a study to record the natural history of syphilis. Originally called the "Tuskegee Study of Untreated Syphilis in the Negro Male". The study involved 600 black men - 400 with syphilis and 200 who did not. Researchers told the men they were being treated for "bad blood," a term used to describe several things such as syphilis, fatigue, anemia.

Syphilis can lead to blindness, deafness, bone deterioration, heart disease, mental illness, the collapse of the central nervous system, and death. In exchange for taking part in the study the men received free meals, free medical exams and burial insurance. The purpose of the study was to observe the effects of syphilis when left untreated to the point of death and autopsy.

Penicillin was widely available and known effective for syphilis by 1943–1944. The study continued withholding it until 1972. Raymond A. Vonderlehr was appointed on-site director of the research program. He advertised spinal taps as a "special free treatment." He also met with local black doctors and asked them to deny treatment to patients in the study. The men were not informed of the nature of the study and the denial of penicillin. The men were not informed of their diagnosis of syphilis. They were given placebos, mercury rubs, salvarsan, injections of neoarsphenamine, bismuth, lumbar punctures for treatment for their "bad blood".

After funding was lost the study went from being six months long to 40 years. It was continued without informing the men that they would never be treated. The study continued under numerous Public Health Services supervisors until 1972. By then 28 patients had died directly from syphilis, 100 died from complications related to syphilis, 40 wives of the patients were infected, and 19 children were born with congenital syphilis. Depending on who you ask.

Nurse Eunice Rivers trained and worked at the Tuskegee Institute. She was recruited at the start of the study to be the main contact with the patients. She played a crucial role in the study, as she was seen as key to gaining the trust of the participants and promoting further participation. As part of "Miss River's Lodge" participants would receive free treatment for minor ailments, free physical exams at Tuskegee University, hot meals on examination days, and free rides to and from the clinic. She was the only staff member to work with the patients for the full 40 years.

In 1966 Peter Buxtun, a venereal-disease investigator in San Francisco sent a letter expressing his concerns about the ethics and morality of the extended Tuskegee study. By this time the CDC controlled the study and reaffirmed the need to continue until its completion in other words until all were dead and autopsied.

The story about the study first broke on July 25th 1972 in the Washington Star by Jean Heller, after Buxton finally went to the press. Senator Edward Kennedy called Congressional hearings, Buxtun testified in those trials. As a result of public outcry the Public Health Services and CDC appointed an ad hoc advisory panel to review their study. The panel found the men agreed to simple things such as examination and treatment and that they were not informed of the actual purpose of the study. The panel determined it was medically unjust and ordered it terminated.

In 1997 President Bill Clinton formally apologized and held a ceremony at the White House for survivors of the study. 5 of the 8 survivors attended the ceremony. The five survivors who attended were Carter Howard, Herman Shaw, Charlie Pollard, Fred Simmons, and Fredrick Moss. The other 3 survivors had family members attend in their name. Ernest Hendon by his brother North Hendon, Sam Doner by his daughter Gwendolyn Cox, and George Key by his grandson Christopher Monroe.

Eugenics Program

The concept of superiority in genetics is not a new theory. All throughout our history there are many counts of similar actions as the Eugenics program. Plutarch in ancient Sparta is the sole account of Gerousia (the council of elders) inspecting proper citizens' children to determine if they were fit to live. Plato held the belief that the state should cautiously monitor and control human reproduction through selective breeding. Royalty for centuries believed and married through selective breeding for "purity" and power. Hitler pushed the idea that the Aryan race was genetically superior to all others and the elimination of "unfit" races.

The British Eugenics Education Society of 1907 and the American Eugenic Society of 1921 are examples of organizations that were formed to win public support and sway opinions on eugenic values in parenthood. Both organizations sought out the support of leading clergymen to help modify their message to meet religious ideals.

Starting in the late 1800s by Sir Francis Galton (a cousin of Charles Darwin), who applied ideas of heredity and selective breeding to humans, influenced by Darwin's work. In the early 1900s two Americans championed his ideas. Harry Laughlin (a former teacher interested in animal breeding) and Charles Davenport (a prominent biologist). Francis defined Eugenics as "the study of agencies under social control that may improve or impair the racial qualities of future generations either physically or mentally." He claimed that health and disease, as well as intellectual and social characteristics were based on heredity and the idea of race.

By the 1920s eugenics had become a global movement becoming popular with the elites and governments. Germany, the United States of America, Great Britain, Mexico, Canada, Italy and others all had forms of eugenics. Economists, public health officials, statisticians, sociologists, social reformers, anthropologists, geneticists, and members of the general public all publicly supported eugenics through a variety of literature. Some of the well-respected figures at the time who supported this belief were the Carnegie family, the Rockefeller family, and U.S. President Woodrow Wilson.

The assumption that all traits are genetically determined led to widespread belief that desirable traits should be "selected". Those with unwanted characteristics should be forcibly sterilized to prevent their contribution to the gene pool. This was encouraged and celebrated through "fitter family" and "better baby" competitions. Each state has their own criteria for which people should be sterilized. Some of the people deemed undeniable were labeled "the feebleminded", "mental defectives", "moral degenerates" and "habitual criminals". The descriptions were oftentimes very vague and biased against marginalized groups such as the poor, immigrants and people with disabilities.

In an infamous case Buck v. Bell judges endorsed the surgical sterilization of Carrie Buck, who was pregnant at the age of 16. She became pregnant after being raped by a relative of her foster parents. Officials at the institution where she was sent to keep her pregnancy secret wanted to sterilize her to prevent her from passing on her perceived feeblemindedness to future generations. The court ruled 8-1 that the state could sterilize her. Justice Oliver Wendell Holmes Jr. stated "It is better for all the world, if instead of waiting to execute degenerate offspring for crime, or to let them starve for their imbecility, society can prevent those who are manifestly unfit from continuing their kind. The principle that sustains compulsory vaccination is broad enough to cover cutting the Fallopian tubes." His infamous ending "Three generations of imbeciles are enough."

Ladies and Gentlemen a Supreme Court Justice, with the support of the Majority, said these words in regards to this case.

The landmark decision helped legitimize roughly 60,000 other forced sterilizations that followed. 20,000 of those 60,000 were in California alone between 1907-1960s. The practices were carried out in tax funded institutions for the disabled and mentally ill, public hospitals. People who had disabilities or mental illnesses were deemed unfit for reproduction.

In 2018 the LA county Board of Supervisors issued a formal apology. "Over 200 women who delivered babies at the Los Angeles County+USC Medical Center, the majority of whom were low income and born in Mexico, were possibly coerced into getting postpartum tubal ligations. At least some of the women were not aware they had been sterilized, and only learned that they had lost their reproductive rights during subsequent doctors' visits. It is significant and necessary to acknowledge the irreparable harm inflicted onto the women who were subjected to these coerced sterilizations at Los Angeles County+USC Medical Center, and to their families."

In some cases women were led to believe the procedures were reversible. In other cases sterilization was performed without adequate understanding and without informed consent. There were even procedures performed on minors as young as 11. Even after legislation designed to protect women from being forcefully sterilized was passed in 1974 the abuse continued.

Some officials and doctors at the IHS appeared to believe that American Indian and other minority women did not have the intelligence to use other methods of birth control. That there were already too many minority individuals causing problems in the nation. During the 1970s, thousands of Indigenous women underwent sterilization procedures, and investigations later raised serious concerns about informed consent practices, coercion, and the extent to which patients fully understood the procedures being performed.

In 1976, a U.S. General Accountability Office (GAO) investigation found four IHS areas were noncompliant with policies regulating consent to sterilization. Senator James Abourezk pointed out that the 3,406 sterilizations that were found would be a startling proportion of Native American women. The report only examined four out of the twelve IHS areas. Attempts to collect the total number of sterilizations that happened during this time differ wildly. The count by the GAO represents a minimum with estimates ranging from 25-50% of Native American women being sterilized from 1970-1976.

In their quest for the perfect society eugenicists labelled many people as “unfit”. By the end of World War I most industrialized countries had organizations devoted to promoting eugenics. This is just a brief summary of what happened. I did not go into details too much on what these women went through. I don't feel I need to. Just knowing there were forced sterilizations tells you everything these women experienced. If you want further details on some of what happened to these women I will simply encourage you to look it up.

Below is a link to the California case. But keep in mind those are only 20,000 of the 60,000 women who were sterilized under state eugenic policies across the United States. This was in the early 1900s to the 1960s some cases into the 1970s. History repeatedly shows that some of humanity's worst mistakes began with people convinced they were improving society. What practices are we currently using today that in just a few years could be deemed horrific?

CIA MKULTRA 1953-1973

Fear of "brain warfare" terrified and fascinated the American public throughout the 1950s. Spurred by stories of "brainwashed" G.I.s returning from Korea, China and the Soviet Union. Headlines like "New Evils Seen in Brainwashing" and "Brainwashing vs Western Psychiatry" didn't help matters either.

During the early 1940s Nazi scientists working in the concentration camps of World War II were conducting interrogation experiments on human subjects. Those subjects were prisoners of war, Polish, Ukrainian, Russian, and Jewish. They were given substances such as morphine derivatives, barbiturates, and hallucinogens such as Mescaline. The goal was to develop a "truth serum" that would "eliminate the will of the person". Mescaline would later become one of several psychoactive substances studied by American intelligence programs, including projects that eventually led to MKUltra.

In 1938 Albert Hofmann at Sandoz Lab in Basel Switzerland isolated LSD. In 1950 the Central Intelligence Agency under the direction of General Walter Bedell Smith initiated a series of interrogation projects involving human subjects. With the launch of Project Bluebird officially renamed Project Artichoke on August 20th 1951. Overseen and directed by Brigadier General Paul F. Gaynor using Mescaline, Morphine, and LSD, administered them to unknowing people with the intent of producing amnesia in subjects. Project Artichoke also aimed to use certain viruses such as Dengue fever as an incapacitating agent.

Project MKUltra started in April 1953, director Sidney Gottlieb arranged for the CIA to buy the entire supply of LSD for $240,000 (today's value is millions). The acquisition gave Gottlieb access to a large supply of LSD for the agency's growing research programs. Along with high doses of LSD they also used other psychoactive drugs and other chemicals. Non-chemical methods that were used were isolation, sensory deprivation, verbal and sexual abuse, hypnosis, electroshocks, and other forms of torture.

MKUltra carried out their activities at more than 80 institutions, hospitals, colleges and universities, pharmaceutical companies, prisons, clinics, foundations and throughout the military all under the guise of research. Researchers involved in MKUltra studied a wide range of topics including interrogation techniques, behavior modification, memory, hypnosis, and the effects of psychoactive drugs on unwitting and willing subjects. Surprise acid trips became an almost occupational hazard for CIA operatives. There was one operative who was drugged in his morning coffee and became psychotic and ran across Washington, D.C. seeing monsters in every passing car.

The CIA wanted to know if they could make Soviet spies defect against their will. Other experiments administered LSD on prisoners, prostitutes, mental patients and drug addicts or "people who could not fight back" as one agent put it. In one case they administered LSD to a mental patient in Kentucky for 174 days. 174 days really think about that! Doctors, government agents, military personnel and members of the general public were also given LSD. Military personnel were threatened with court-martial if they said anything about the experiments. Some researchers hoped to find ways to erase memories, increase compliance, extract information, or create individuals who could unknowingly carry out instructions. Internal documents reveal that some proposals bordered on ideas that today sound more like science fiction than medicine. Governments have spent how much money to come up with a "super soldier"?

Ready for a rather bizarre aspect of these operations? Through Operation Midnight Climax, the CIA set up several brothels within agency safehouses in San Francisco, CA. To obtain a group of men who would be too embarrassed to talk afterwards. The men were dosed with LSD, agents filmed through one-way mirrors so they could view and study later. In other experiments people were given LSD without knowledge, then interrogated with bright lights while doctors took notes. Some of the people subjected to these experiments were U.S. military personnel and CIA agents suspected of working for the Soviet Block during the Cold War.

The CIA using a front called the Society for the Investigation of Human Ecology, hired a Scottish psychiatrist Donald Ewen Cameron living in Canada. Cameron is the creator of the concept "psychic driving" which the CIA found interesting. Cameron hoped to fix schizophrenia by erasing memories and reprogramming the psyche. Internal CIA documents showed Cameron was unaware the money was coming from the CIA. He did his experiments at Allan Memorial Institute of McGill University in Montreal Canada from 1957-1964 (some suggest it starting as early as 1948).

Cameron experimented on patients using LSD, electroconvulsive therapy at higher than normal power, as well as various paralytic drugs. His "driving" experiments put subjects into drug induced comas for weeks, three months in one case. Tapes on loop playing noise or repetitive statements were played while they were in the coma. Often his subjects were patients who came in the institute for common problems like postpartum depression or anxiety disorders. His treatments often led to amnesia, forgetting how to talk, urinary incontinence, thinking interrogators were their parents, forgetting their family members. Cameron was a member of the Nuremberg medical tribunal in 1946-1947. During the time of his experiments he became known worldwide as president of both the Canadian and American Psychiatric Association as well as the first chairman of the World Psychiatric Association.

In 1973 during the panic of the Watergate scandal the then CIA Director Richard Helms ordered MKUltra files be destroyed. Due to this order, doing a full investigation into the more than 150 funded research subprojects and related CIA programs was difficult. In December of 1974, The New York Times alleged that the CIA had conducted illegal domestic activities including experimenting on U.S. citizens during the 1960s. Due to their allegations the U.S. congress using the Church Committee with the Rockefeller Commission began looking into illegal domestic activities of the CIA, FBI and other intelligence related agencies within the military.

Luckily 20,000 documents survived because they were incorrectly stored in a financial records building. They were discovered following a FOIA request in Senate Hearings of 1977. Those surviving documents were fully investigated during the hearings. Cameron died on September 8th, 1967, none of his personal records of his involvement in MKUltra survived. His family destroyed them after his death. A 1986 report found that Canadian government officials were not fully aware of his experiments.

During a hearing by the Senate Health Subcommittee a testimony by the deputy director of the CIA stated that 30 institutions and universities were involved in the experimentation program. They were testing drugs and other studies on unknowing citizens "at all social levels, high and low, native Americans and foreign." The Army was subject to testing of LSD in three phases. First was 1,000 soldiers who volunteered for testing of chemical warfare experiments. The second phase had 96 volunteers who were dosed with LSD to see the possibility of intelligence uses of the drug. The third and final was Project Third Chance and Project Derby Hat which experimented on 16 unknowing non-volunteer subjects that received LSD and then were interrogated for hours. Many of those veterans later sought legal and monetary reparations.

In 1976 President Gerald Ford issued an Executive Order on Intelligence Activities. Part of the order prohibited "experimentation with drugs on human subjects, except with the informed consent, in writing and witnessed by a disinterested party, of each such human subject." President Reagan and President Carter both issued orders expanding the directive to apply to any human experimentation. In 1985 CIA v. Sims, The U.S. Supreme Court endorsed mosaic effect to justify broad judicial deference under FOIA Exemption 3. This enabled the CIA to withhold details about MKUltra because disclosures could expose intelligence sources.

Ladies and gentlemen, for years intelligence agencies secretly conducted experiments on unwitting individuals, often without informed consent and sometimes with little regard for the consequences. Remember this all happened in the 60s. What experiments could be going on today that we won't know about until years after? Does it sound familiar to anything else in history? For so many years governments have hid things from their citizens until after the damage has already been done. Far too many times the ones who cause the damage aren't justly convicted.

Operation Paperclip / Overcast / Cover-up of Unit 731

In order to understand the gravity of what Operation Paperclip did you need to know what happened to the victims. There is heavy debate even today over the exact number of people who fell victim to the human experimentations of World War II. Honestly the numbers aren't the important part, it's what happened to these people that really matters. We owe these victims remembrance. Some knowledge was gained from the suffering they endured, but that knowledge came at a horrific human cost. The victims paid the price, not by choice, but because it was forced upon them. The use of chemical and biological warfare cost countless soldiers and citizens their lives across numerous countries.

Operation Paperclip was a secret United States of America intelligence program where 1,600 German engineers, technicians and scientists and their families were taken from former Nazi Germany to the U.S. for employment after the end of World War II between 1945 and 1959. Several were confirmed to be former members of the Nazi Party. The US Joint Chiefs of Staff officially established Operation Overcast on July 20th, 1945. Overcast and Paperclip are often used interchangeably.

The operation was largely carried out by special agents of the US Army's Counterintelligence Corps. Many of the selected scientists were involved in the Nazi rocket program, chemical/biological warfare or aviation. The Soviet Union in the following year conducted a similar program called Operation Osoaviakhim. Operation Paperclip relocated more than 1,500 experts to the US.

Those recruited were instrumental in the development of the US space program and military technology during the Cold War. Leading to billions in patents and industrial processes. In the early 1950s Wernher von Braun's team developed Redstone and Jupiter missiles. When the team was transferred to NASA in 1960 it became central to the work of the Marshall Space Flight Center and the development of the Saturn launch vehicles used in the Apollo program. No evidence has linked von Braun to the medical experiments discussed here, though historians continue to debate the extent of his knowledge of and responsibility for the use of forced labor in the German rocket program.

For 50 years from 1963-2013 the most prestigious award from the Space Medicine Association was named after "the father of space medicine" Hubertus Strughold. Strughold played a central role in developing things like the space suit and space life support systems. In early 1944 Strughold was named Aviation Medical Consultant to the new chief of staff of Luftwaffe Medical Service Oskar Schröder. In July 1944 Schröder initiated human experiments at Dachau, one of the first concentration camps built in Nazi Germany.

The study centered on testing new methods of converting seawater to fresh water. 90 Romani inmates were deprived of food and forced to consume large amounts of seawater or had it directly injected into their veins. Half were given a drug called Berkatit and all were forced to endure a liver biopsy without anesthetic. Numerous subjects lost their lives. How much Strughold was aware of or involved in the many war crimes committed at Dachau still remains controversial. An article written in the Wall Street Journal published on December 1st, 2012 highlighted his connection to human experiments during WWII.

Though most of the scientists were never convicted of any crimes, many were members of the Nazi Party. A few like Hubertus Strughold held close ties to connections to war crimes. Only one was formally charged, Georg Rickhey, with accusations that he worked closely with the SS and Gestapo and witnessed executions. Arrested in 1945 he was brought to Wright-Patterson Air Force Base in Ohio

There under Operation Paperclip he helped establish a smuggling operation using knowledge of black markets he gained while in Nazi Germany. Rickhey was accused of hanging 12 prisoners from a crane; he was acquitted due to lack of evidence. He returned to Wright-Patt after the trial but did not rejoin Operation Paperclip.

As we all know there was more than one country involved in the war. These examples from Operation Paperclip are of the Germans that were recruited. Now let's discuss how far the U.S. Government went to help cover up the crimes of Unit 731 in Japan.

The US government sent General MacArthur to oversee the rebuilding of post war Japan. During the occupation, MacArthur assigned a Lieutenant Colonel Murray Sanders to gather information on Japan's "biological warfare", aka the information gathered through their human experimentation. U.S. occupation authorities ultimately granted immunity to several Unit 731 leaders in exchange for access to data gathered through the program's experiments.

In September 1945 Officer General Shirō Ishii and General Masaji Kitano (of Unit 731) were pardoned for their role in Japanese war crimes. While a series of war tribunals and trials were being organized the US government classified incriminating evidence as well as blocked the prosecution's access to key witnesses, in order to pardon many of the high ranking officials and doctors who planned and performed the experiments. Estimates of the total number of victims vary widely among historians, ranging from hundreds of thousands to more than half a million people affected by Unit 731, Unit 100, and related biological warfare activities.

The atrocities of Unit 731 should have never been forgiven. Unit 731's activities included infecting prisoners with deadly diseases, organ harvesting, amputating limbs, testing hypobaric chambers, conducting vivisection, exposing victims to chemical agents and explosives. Prisoners were mainly Chinese civilians, but also among them were Russians, Koreans and others including pregnant women and children. That was just within the facilities, they are also responsible for contaminating water, food supply and agricultural land affecting the lives of people in Chinese cities and villages near Manchuria.

One of the experiments that is talked about most comes from an experiment run by General Ishii. The prisoners were infected with disease-causing agents and exposed to bombs that released infectious substances on contact with the skin. Anyone who survived the infection was murdered for autopsy analysis. After experimenting on the prisoners researchers commonly used chloroform or potassium cyanide to kill them. A few things they were infected with are venereal diseases such as syphilis, gonorrhea.

Prisoners were referred to as "logs" due to the cover story for the facility being a lumber mill. A common phrase referencing how many prisoners died was "How many logs fell?". Prisoners were held in facilities called "log cabins". The corpses were disposed of by incineration.

Hideo Shimizu at the age of 14 along with 34 boys around his age made up the 4th group of minors that were assigned to Unit 731. For the first few days they were told to memorize "Senjinjkun" (instructions for the battlefield), a military code that stated, "Never live to experience shame as a prisoner." Shimizu was assigned to an education department laboratory where he studied pathogens and how to cultivate them. His every movement and conversations were heavily restricted. Shimizu talks about the nightmares he has of what he calls the specimen room.

The specimen room was lined with jars filled with human remains preserved in formalin. There were heads, hands, other human body parts and one contained a pregnant woman with the lower part of her belly cut open to display a fetus with hair. Shimizu was also ordered to pick up the bones of prisoners. The Russians invaded only a few short months after he was sent there.

At the age of 93 while visiting a museum about Unit 731 Shimizu shared his experience with his wife for the very first time. He tried to publicly share his story causing people to call him a liar. Discussions floating around at the time called Unit 731 a hoax, there was even a book written. In May of 2022 a peace memorial museum opened in Ida, a Nagano Prefecture Japan. It was expected to feature testimonies by Shimizu on a panel about Unit 731. It was abandoned by the city's board of education which runs the museum. Stating it needed to carefully consider the issue because academic research is still being conducted on Unit 731 and due to diverse opinions on the matter in society.

The brutality of the human experimentations that were conducted during WWII are still hard for people to learn about. The full scope of what occurred during these programs continues to be studied and debated, particularly regarding the total number of victims and the long-term impact of the research. The atrocities themselves, however, remain among the darkest documented chapters of the war. This is not the only time in our history when the government helped the criminal. This is not the only time that "dark secrets" were buried and hidden from the public. How many more were buried that we don't have any idea about? How many are currently going on that we may never know about?

Want to Dig Deeper?

The following pages contain links to museum collections, archives, historical photographs, public records, documentaries, and other resources related to each section of this book.

Scan the QR code or type the web address to continue your investigation.

Forced Sterilization of Native American Women

Explore:

https://daily.jstor.org/the-little-known-history-of-the-forced-sterilization-of-native-american-women/

The Tuskegee Syphilis Study

Explore:

https://historycollection.com/20-photos-tuskegee-syphilis-study/

Unit 731

Explore:

https://www.pacificatrocities.org/blog/immunity-for-atrocity-the-us-cover-up-of-unit-731-and-the-corruption-of-postwar-bioethics

Eugenics

Explore:

https://fee.org/articles/a-brief-history-of-california-s-eugenics-program-1909-2013/

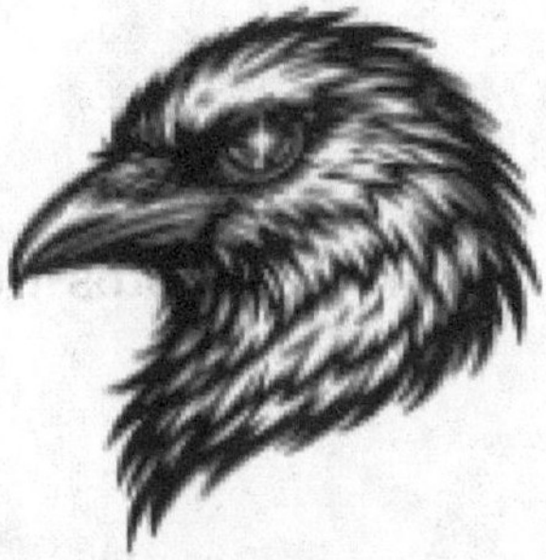

The Questions Remain

We have reached the end of this journey, but the questions do not end here.

Throughout these pages we have explored ideas that were once treated as established facts. We examined skulls drilled in the name of healing, blood drained in the name of medicine, women diagnosed for emotions that are now considered part of being human, and entire groups of people labeled defective, dangerous, or diseased because they challenged the beliefs of their time.

We looked at governments that concealed information, institutions that protected themselves, experts who were convinced they were right, and ordinary people who suffered the consequences when they were wrong.

Some of these stories are centuries old. Others occurred within living memory. Yet they all share a common thread: people rarely recognize they are standing on unstable ground while they are standing on it.

History is filled with individuals who were certain.

Certain the earth worked a particular way.

Certain a treatment was beneficial.

Certain a group of people was inferior.

Certain a diagnosis was legitimate.

Certain a policy served the greater good.

Again and again, time revealed cracks in those certainties.

That realization should not leave us cynical.

It should leave us humble.

For all of humanity's mistakes, there is another side to these stories. We learned. We improved. We questioned old assumptions. We abandoned ideas that caused suffering. Progress did not come from blind acceptance. It came from people willing to challenge what everyone else believed to be true.

That process never ends.

The purpose of this book was never to provide all the answers. Quite the opposite. It was written as an invitation to question, to investigate, and to look beyond the surface of the stories we are told. The official version is often only the beginning. There are always details left out, perspectives forgotten, records buried, and lessons waiting to be rediscovered.

Somewhere in these pages, I hope you found at least one question that refuses to leave you alone.

Follow it.

Pull the thread.

See where it leads.

Read the sources. Challenge the assumptions. Question the experts, but also question yourself. Be willing to change your mind when the evidence demands it. The goal is not to distrust everything. The goal is to understand more than you did yesterday.

The past is not dead. It echoes through every institution, belief, law, and tradition we inherit. Its lessons remain available to anyone willing to listen.

So as you close this book, I leave you with the same challenge that inspired its creation:

What are we absolutely certain about today that future generations may one day question?

Whatever answer comes to mind, start there.

Stay curious.

Stay humble.

Never stop digging.

The rabbit holes are waiting.

Willow Ravencrest

APPENDIX

A. **Timeline of Topics Covered in order as they appear in the book:**

• 6500 BCE – Evidence of trephination (skull drilling) in France and other ancient societies

• Ancient Times (~1900 BCE onward) – Diagnosis of Hysteria ("wandering womb")

• 1692–1693 – Salem Witch Trials (part of centuries-long European Witch Hunts)

• 1796 – Franz Joseph Gall introduces Phrenology

• Early 1800s – Bloodletting widely used as a standard medical treatment

• 1835 – James Cowles Prichard defines "Moral Insanity"

• 1840s – Ignaz Semmelweis fights for handwashing

• 1851 – Samuel Cartwright coins "Drapetomania"

• Early 1900s – "Cure" for left-handedness commonly practiced on children

• 1910s–1920s – The Radium Girls tragedy

• 1920s–1960s – Smoking advertised as healthy by doctors and companies

• 1930s–1960s – Transorbital Lobotomy of Walter Freeman II

• 1932–1972 – Tuskegee Syphilis Study

• 1945–1959 – Operation Paperclip

• 1945–1948 – U.S. immunity agreements involving Unit 731 personnel

• 1953–1973 – CIA MKUltra experiments

• 1960s–1976 – Forced sterilizations of Native American women

• 1960s-1990s – Sluggish schizophrenia

• Late 1800s – 1970s – Eugenics movement / forced sterilizations in the U.S.

• 1980s–1990s – Satanic Panic & Recovered Memory Therapy

• Early 1900s – Early 2000s – Homo Conversion Therapy

• Ancient Times – Present – Mental disorders, asylums, and treatments

• 1990s–Present – Gulf War Syndrome and ongoing veteran struggles

B. **Expanded Glossary**

Phrenology: The pseudoscience of assessing personality, intelligence, and character by measuring bumps and shapes on a person's skull.

Trephination (Trepanation): The ancient practice of drilling or cutting a hole into the skull, sometimes to treat head injuries, epilepsy, or spiritual issues.

Bloodletting: The intentional removal of blood (using leeches, cuts, or cups) to supposedly restore balance in the body.

Hysteria: A now-discredited medical diagnosis, primarily for women, once believed to be caused by a "wandering womb."

Moral Insanity: A 19th-century diagnosis for people who behaved immorally or antisocially without showing obvious intellectual impairment.

Drapetomania: A racist pseudodiagnosis claiming that enslaved Black people who tried to escape were suffering from a mental illness.

Sluggish Schizophrenia: A Soviet-era diagnosis used to label and institutionalize political dissidents who showed no clear psychotic symptoms.

Lobotomy: A procedure that surgically severs connections in the brain's frontal lobes, often leaving patients severely impaired.

Radium Jaw (Radium Necrosis): severe destruction of the jawbone caused by prolonged radium exposure.

Eugenics: The now-discredited belief that the human population could (and should) be "improved" through selective breeding and forced sterilization.

Conversion Therapy: Attempts to change a person's sexual orientation or gender identity, often using harmful psychological or physical methods.

Recovered Memory Therapy: A controversial technique that claimed to help patients recover repressed memories, later widely criticized for creating false memories.

Mass Hysteria: A phenomenon in which groups of people experience shared fears, beliefs, or physical symptoms that spread through social influence rather than an identifiable physical cause.

MKUltra: Secret CIA research program that conducted illegal mind-control and behavior modification experiments, often using LSD and psychological manipulation.

Operation Paperclip: The U.S. government program that recruited Nazi scientists and engineers after World War II.

Unit 731: A Japanese biological and chemical warfare unit during WWII responsible for horrific human experiments.

Pseudoscience: Claims or practices presented as scientific but lacking proper evidence, testing, or scientific validity.

Puerperal Fever: A life-threatening infection in women after childbirth, also known as childbed fever.

C. **Suggested Reading**

If a particular topic sparked your curiosity, these books offer an excellent place to continue exploring.

No single book can tell the whole story. These works represent a variety of researchers, historians, and perspectives. Whenever possible, compare sources, examine the evidence for yourself, and continue asking questions.

Medical Ethics & Human Experimentation

Medical Apartheid by Harriet A. Washington

Bad Blood: The Tuskegee Syphilis Experiment by James H. Jones

The Radium Girls by Kate Moore

Eugenics & Forced Sterilization

Imbeciles: The Supreme Court, American Eugenics, and the Sterilization of Carrie Buck by Adam Cohen

War Against the Weak: Eugenics and America's Campaign to Create a Master Race by Edwin Black

Mind Control & Intelligence Programs
Poisoner in Chief: Sidney Gottlieb and the CIA Search for Mind Control by Stephen Kinzer

Acid Dreams: The Complete Social History of LSD by Martin A. Lee & Bruce Shlain

Psychiatry & Lobotomy

The Lobotomist: A Maverick Medical Genius and His Tragic Quest to Rid the World of Mental Illness by Jack El-Hai

My Lobotomy by Howard Dully

World War II & Government Secrecy

Operation Paperclip: The Secret Intelligence Program That Brought Nazi Scientists to America by Annie Jacobsen

SUGGESTED BIBLIOGRAPHY

A Note on the Sources

The sources listed here represent only a small portion of the material consulted while researching this book.

Many chapters required reviewing historical documents, academic journals, government reports, court records, newspaper archives, books, museum collections, and other primary and secondary sources. Including every source would add dozens of additional pages.

History is rarely told through a single voice. Whenever possible, I encourage you to read original documents, compare multiple perspectives, and continue exploring these topics for yourself. Curiosity doesn't end with this book—it begins here.

The Radium Girls by Kate Moore (already in your list – the definitive book on the subject)

Bad Blood: The Tuskegee Syphilis Experiment by James H. Jones

Imbeciles: The Supreme Court, American Eugenics, and the Sterilization of Carrie Buck by Adam Cohen

War Against the Weak: Eugenics and America's Campaign to Create a Master Race by Edwin Black

Operation Paperclip: The Secret Intelligence Program That Brought Nazi Scientists to America by Annie Jacobsen

Poisoner in Chief: Sidney Gottlieb and the CIA Search for Mind Control by Stephen Kinzer (excellent on MKUltra)

Acid Dreams: The Complete Social History of LSD by Martin A. Lee and Bruce Shlain

The Lobotomist: A Maverick Medical Genius and His Tragic Quest to Rid the World of Mental Illness by Jack El-Hai

Medical Apartheid: The Dark History of Medical Experimentation on Black Americans by Harriet A. Washington

My Lobotomy by Howard Dully (a powerful firsthand survivor account)

Articles & Reports

U.S. General Accountability Office. Report on Sterilizations at Indian Health Service Facilities. Washington, DC: GAO, 1976.

Websites & Online Sources

British Museum. "Everything You Ever Wanted to Know About the Rosetta Stone." The British Museum Blog. https://www.britishmuseum.org/blog/everything-you-ever-wanted-know-about-rosetta-stone.

Deanna Dupont. "Moral Insanity Part 2 of 3." Substack, n.d. https://deannadupont.substack.com/p/moral-insanity-part-2-of-3.

Digital Public Library of America. "The Invention of the Telephone." https://dp.la/primary-source-sets/the-invention of-the-telephone.

Foundation for Economic Education. "A Brief History of California's Eugenics Program (1909–2013)." https://fee.org/articles/a-brief-history-of-california-s-eugenics-program-1909-2013/.

Go2Tutors. "15 Forgotten Toys That Were Pulled for Being Too Weird." https://go2tutors.com/15-forgotten-toys-that-were-pulled-for-being-too-weird.

History Collection. "20 Photos from the Tuskegee Syphilis Study." https://historycollection.com/20-photos-tuskegee-syphilis-study/.

Library of Congress. "Who Is Credited with Inventing the Telephone?" Everyday Mysteries. https://www.loc.gov/everyday-mysteries/technology/item/who-is-credited-with-inventing-the-telephone/.

National Center for Biotechnology Information. "The Lobotomy Patient—A Decade Later: A Follow-up Study of a Research Project Started in 1948." https://pmc.ncbi.nlm.nih.gov/articles/PMC1922743/.

Pacific Atrocities. "Immunity for Atrocity: The US Cover-Up of Unit 731." https://www.pacificatrocities.org/blog/immunity-for-atrocity-the-us-cover-up-of-unit-731-and-the-corruption-of-postwar-bioethics.

Public Domain Review. "Phrenology Diagrams from Vaught's Practical Character Reader (1902)." https://publicdomainreview.org/collection/phrenology-diagrams-from-vaught-s-practical-character-reader-1902/.

Rare Historical Photos. "Bizarre Vintage Tobacco Advertising." https://rarehistoricalphotos.com/bizarre-vintage-tobacco-advertising/.

Science History Institute. "Ignaz Semmelweis." https://www.sciencehistory.org/education/scientific-biographies/ignaz-semmelweis/.

Wikimedia Commons. "Trephined Skull." By Anagoria. CC BY 3.0. https://commons.wikimedia.org/w/index.php?curid=26657586.

Wood Library-Museum of Anesthesiology. "History of Anesthesia." https://www.woodlibrarymuseum.org/history-of-anesthesia/.

World History Encyclopedia. "The Printing Revolution in Renaissance Europe." https://www.worldhistory.org/article/

1632/the-printing-revolution-in-renaissance-europe/.

ABOUT THE AUTHOR

Willow Ravencrest is an independent author whose work explores the forgotten corners of history, psychology, science, and human behavior. Drawn to the uncomfortable questions many people overlook, she enjoys digging beneath accepted narratives to examine how beliefs evolve, how mistakes become normalized, and how today's certainties may become tomorrow's curiosities.

Curious Atrocities: The Dark Side of Obscured History is her first published nonfiction work. Rather than offering final answers, Willow hopes to inspire readers to think critically, compare sources, and continue asking questions long after they turn the final page.

When she isn't disappearing down historical rabbit holes, she is developing future nonfiction projects and writing fantasy novels.
"
Curiosity is rarely comfortable—but it is often where discovery begins."

CALL TO ACTION

If this book has left you unsettled, curious, surprised, or even frustrated, then it has accomplished exactly what I hoped it would.

History is rarely as simple as we are taught. The deeper we dig, the more we discover that many of humanity's greatest mistakes were made by people who believed they were absolutely certain they were right.

Now the journey becomes yours.

Don't let this book be the end of your curiosity. Let it be the beginning.

Read beyond these pages. Explore the sources. Compare different perspectives. Seek out original documents whenever you can. Ask difficult questions—even of ideas you already agree with. Some rabbit holes will confirm what you believe. Others may completely change your mind. Both are valuable.

If you enjoyed this book, consider sharing it with someone else who loves asking questions and exploring the forgotten corners of history. An honest review is also one of the greatest gifts you can give an independent author, helping other curious readers discover this work.

Above all else, remember this:

Stay curious.

Stay humble.

Keep asking better questions.

Because knowledge is never finished. Every generation uncovers forgotten stories, challenges old assumptions, and discovers that certainty is often temporary.

The rabbit holes are endless.

The next one is waiting.

WILLOW RAVENCREST

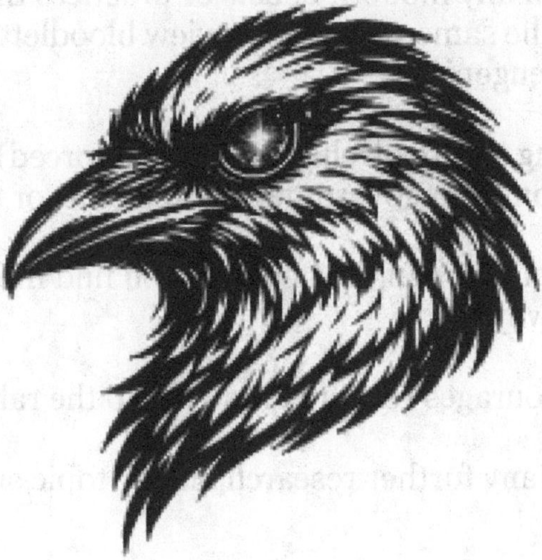

Book Club Questions

Reader's Discussion Guide:

This book is designed to spark conversation and critical thinking. Here are some questions to help you reflect on the material — whether you're reading alone or discussing it with a group.

Discussion Questions:

Which chapter or topic surprised you the most? Why?

Were there any topics in this book that made you uncomfortable? What does that discomfort tell you?

The author argues that we must face ugly truths in order to grow. Do you agree? Why or why not?

Can you think of any modern beliefs or practices that might one day be viewed the same way we now view bloodletting, lobotomies, or eugenics?

How has reading this book changed (or reinforced) the way you view information from governments, medicine, or media?

Which historical figure in the book did you find most tragic or inspiring, and why?

The author encourages readers to "step into the rabbit holes."

Have you done any further research on any topic since reading this book?

How should we balance skepticism with trust in institutions (science, government, medicine)?

Do you believe society has genuinely learned from past mistakes, or do similar patterns continue today in different forms?

If you could add one more chapter to this book, what topic would you want the author to explore next?

How has this book affected the way you talk to your children or younger family members about history?

What is one practical way you can apply the lessons from this book in your daily life?

Final Reflection Question:

What is one belief you once held strongly that you later discovered was wrong? How did that realization change you?

For Those of You Who Found This, Welcome to the Easter Egg!

In this section I'm not going to go into too much detail about these discoveries, instead I will ask something of you dear reader. Go to the suggested links and check them out for yourself. Some you may find mind numbingly boring but some you may find draw you in and fascinate you. As you go though these keep one thing in mind, all of these changed the way the world viewed something big. It opened a massive group of people's eyes to a completely different way of seeing the world. It also proved that our previous ways of thinking were wrong. That ladies and gentlemen is what it's all about, how you grow from your flaws. Can you admit there was a mistake, so that you can learn a new way of thinking? Life is about constantly growing and evolving internally and physically. Just like how these discoveries changed the way the world thought and looked.

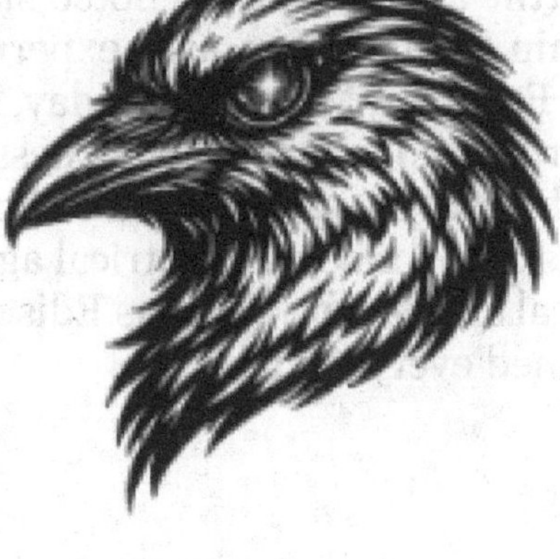

Rosetta Stone-

A stele/slab of granodiorite inscribed with 3 versions of a decree issued in 196 BC on behalf of King PtolemyV Epiphanes. The top two texts are in Ancient Egyptian
Hieroglyphics and Demotic scripts, the third on the bottom was in Ancient Greek. It became key in deciphering Egyptian scripts that before were unknown or guessed at. In July 1799 a French army officer Pierre-Francois Bouchard discovered it while rebuilding Fort Julien near port city Rosetta (present-day Rashid). It now sits in a British museum.

https://www.britishmuseum.org/blog/everything-you-ever-wanted-know-about-rosetta-stone

Discovery of Gravity-

Isaac Newton, a mathematician and physicist discovered gravity at the age of 23. Newton's works and understanding of gravity are used to explain from the trajectory of a ball to the Earth's orbit around the sun. He also later published a book "Principia" which explained his 3 laws of motion as well as expanding on his laws of universal gravitation. His work laid the foundations of modern day physics.

Discovery of Electricity-

Electricity was observed and studied for centuries before the 18th and 19th centuries (the ancient Greeks noted static electricity with amber, and Benjamin Franklin famously experimented with his kite in 1752). Benjamin Franklin, Michael Faraday, and James Clerk Maxwell began to truly understand and harness electricity. Faraday's work with electromagnetism and Maxwell's equations laid the foundations of the modern electrical age. With the invention of practical systems by Thomas Edison and Nikola Tesla, electricity transformed everyday life.

The Printing Press

Invented in the 15th century the printing press by Johannes Gutenberg. With his invention books could be mass produced. Before they were copied by hand which made knowledge scarce and expensive. It fueled education, spread scientific knowledge and fueled the renaissance and Enlightenment. Knowledge became readily available to the average person. Reading and writing became a norm instead of something that was only for the wealthy.

https://www.worldhistory.org/article/1632/the-printing revolution-in-renaissance-europe/

Anesthesia

It wasn't until the 19th century when doctors began using chloroform to knock people unconscious during surgery. Later more effective and safer anesthetics were created. Before this patients would be fully awake relying on opium, alcohol, or brute force to get them through. It expanded what types of procedures were possible, made surgery more humane, and saved countless lives.

https://www.woodlibrarymuseum.org/history-of-anesthesia/

The Telephone

1876 Alexander Graham Bell invented the telephone, changing how the world communicates. It connected families over vast distances, helped facilitate business, and transformed emergency response. Becoming what we now hold in our hands every day, the modern cell phone.

https://www.loc.gov/everyday-mysteries/technology/item/who-is-credited-with-inventing-the-telephone/

https://dp.la/primary-source-sets/the-invention-of-the-telephone#tabs

Toys Removed from the Market

Over the years there have been a many toys that were removed from the market for various reasons. Some for choking hazards others for danger risks. As we progress into the modern era where the internet, cameras and microphones and now AI are making their way into toys. Who knows how many toys will be removed from the market in a few years or how many more risky toys will make their way onto the market.

https://doyouremember.com/1553/dangerous-toys-that-were-pulled-off-the-market

https://go2tutors.com/15-forgotten-toys-that-were-pulled-for-being-too-weird/

www.ingramcontent.com/pod-product-compliance
Lightning Source LLC
LaVergne TN
LVHW030727061126
851857LV00019B/2027
* 9 7 9 8 2 3 4 1 5 5 8 0 1 *